MISCELLANEOUS

MEMOIRS

OF THE MAD

Book description

"In the cold clockworks of the stars and the nations, the warping of the space continuum, and the depths of natural galaxies (as humans), we are, in all candour, significantly insignificant, burdened with idle purpose. We are ailed with internal suffering. I am not fooled by the façade of hope, nor the mirage of a future. I wish to deposit my packages of pain."

This was the bitterly hopeless words of a suicidal with Emotionally Unstable Personality Disorder, attachment issues, autism, depression and psychosis, stuck in 8 different secure psychiatric units over the course of 4 years as a teenager.

Listen to the story of a girl who was running into walls, thinking that they were portals; had to get people to taste-test food because she thought it was contaminated with poison or trackers, was nursed by having 3 staff members stay with me at all times (even on the toilet) to restrain me from hurting myself or others.

But this also includes a girl who was chased by a psychotic boy who was naked and was drenched in his own poo; asked Santa for sweets for the "psych ward around the corner" and pranked a fully grown registered mental health nurse into believing there was a snake in the secure garden of the psychiatric intensive care unit.

Follow me on my journey which broke me and shattered every last shred of hope which eventually led to my gradual, painfully slow process of rebuilding the foundations to my mind. I fixed myself. I now give lectures about my experience to share my journey, working towards my education and have worked hard for a life worth living.

I overcame wanting to die by learning how to want to live. I survived. This is the story of an ex-suicidal.

DISCLAIMER:

I have tried to recreate events, locales and conversations from my memories of them. In order to maintain their anonymity in some instances I have changed the names of individuals and places, I may have changed some identifying characteristics and details such as physical properties, occupations and places of residence. Please note that this is based off real life events.

This book is not intended as a substitute for the medical advice of physicians. The reader should regularly consult a physician in matters relating to his/her health and particularly with respect to any symptoms that may require diagnosis or medical attention.

Any reference to fictional places or names are not owned by me, nor am I liable for legal disciplinary action for mention of them. They are used as terms of reference only.

This disclaimer informs readers that the views, thoughts, and opinions expressed in the text belong solely to the author, and not necessarily to the author's employer, organization, committee or other group or individual.

Trigger warning: there is mention of self-harm and suicide. However great caution was taken in order to remove any methodical implications of these themes. This could be distressing to some readers.

To all People who are struggling,

You were given this life because you are strong enough to live it. The world is a better place with you in it.

Thank you to all the people I have met on my journey, I wouldn't be alive without you.

Preface:

My name is ZeZe Jones. I am an 18 year old who likes unicorns, make-up, studying and the gym. I am a normal person...whatever "normal" is. Except I have suffered with poor mental health for 7 years. And I was sectioned over the course of 4 years. It challenged me, it changed me. After nearly losing my life on multiple occasions, here I am sharing my journey. I made it. I made it because the fire in me burned brighter than the fire around me. I decided that my story wasn't finished yet. I chose recovery.

Whether you are someone struggling with their mental health, a professional or someone else, here is my lived experience.

Please listen to the story of an ex-suicidal.

Phase 1: Miscellaneous Journey to Recovery: Was this the end or was it just the beginning?

Chapter 1

Mental Health Hospitals

Mental institution. Sanitarium. Crazy asylum. People automatically think of people struggling in straitjackets with a muzzle over their mouth and a wild, unhinged look in their eye, all whilst being strapped to a bed. Everybody assumes that hospital is only for serial killers and, to put it colloquially, "whackerdoodles who are totes cray-cray". It's supposedly an ersatz environment-called "low-stimulus" -where even the childhood comfort of teddy bears are risk-assessed) for the delusional or criminally insane. Those of whom are restrained by men in white nursing uniforms, held down against their will to endure electroshock therapy, at least once a week. A top psychiatrist will have you speak with them to formulae a psychoanalysis and it is up to them, and them only, to set you free. These psychiatrists will attempt to persuade you to believe that you are unwell- what utter blarney: my voices told me I am sane. You are detached from "the real world" with an abundance of white masked doors standing between you and your way out, a hindrance to the exit. Indestructible metal bars like the windows and every single crevice. Even the sunlight is afraid to spill through the reinforced glass. Food is served through the hole in the door and you are disappointed to have been handed some mushy, unknown slobbery substance which is arguably a source of sustenance. You are forcefully given any psychotropic available, from antipsychotics to sedatives, where they are injected into your bum cheek every day. There is a wide variety of dysthymics, who sit quietly, silently troubled by the world around; manic individuals dancing on table tops; schizophrenics writing conspiracy theories on their wall; and don't forget the catatonics.

As you walk into a bare room with simply a mattress, your roommate whispers, sneering in your ear, "Good night, sleep tight. Don't let the psych patients bite!" There is a phalanx of patients all united for one common reason: detention under the mental health act, in other words, deemed clinically crazy and shunned by society.

"What utter blarney- my voices told me I am sane", they say.

This is the perception of many members of the public, wrongly gained, due to the inaccurate portrayal of mental health by media. People with mental illness do not deserve to put in the metaphorical box of "Crazy". There is so much more to us than that. We are more than our mental illness. This propaganda about mental health is unjustified. It is not even a stigma-I would go as far as to call it discrimination! This is not an accurate representation of being mentally ill- so let me show you what is.

People don't wear muzzles and straitjackets these days. The most abstruse items of clothing they would wear is non-rip, anti-ligature clothing to keep themselves safe if they are at risk of harming themselves. Nobody gets strapped to beds; it is against human rights. Hospital is not just for serial killers. It is full of people who are unwell and need further intensive support. Serial killers go to maximum high-secure forensic psychiatric units. Most people who go to hospital for psychiatric treatment, go to an open rehabilitation unit. If this isn't suitable, there are more specialised units, dependent on risk, type of illness and compliance with treatment.

For adolescents, this is how the mental health inpatient system goes:

General Adolescent Unit

(GAU)

Also called "open/acute" ward.

Where someone goes if they need an inpatient bed but it isn't secure and the doors are not always locked.

I spent 4 months in one GAU and 3 months in another but my risk couldn't be managed on here so I was transferred.

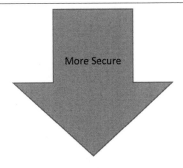

More Secure

High Dependency Unit (HDU)

A ward which is always locked and has plastic cutlery. Meant to be a short stay ward. More secure than GAU but not as secure as Psychiatric Intensive Care Unit.

I had 3 admissions to an HDU. The first was 9 months, the second was 2 months, third was 4 months.

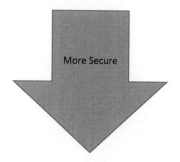

More Secure

Psychiatric Intensive Care Unit (PICU)

A really secure environment where most rooms are locked, there is plastic cutlery, there is a seclusion room where it is completely sterile to keep risky behaviours contained.

It is supposed to be a really short stay ward; either you are there 2- 4 weeks to stabilise the young person or longer if they require further assessment.

There is no facility to have long term stays or long term therapy.

For most people who come here, it is as a last resort. All people here on a section.

If the patient is well enough, they could be discharged or sent to a GAU. If not, will stay in the PICU or go to a Low Secure Unit.

A lot of people in PICUs are there for Drug-Induced Psychosis or are suicidal.

I was in my first PICU for 3 weeks and my second one was for 3 months.

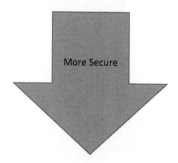

More Secure

Low Secure Unit (LSU)

A really secure unit to manage severe self-harm. Some people who come here come for long term therapy because it is a long term hospital.

Most people who come here on a section 3 which lasts for 6 months, then renewed for a year, then 2 years at a time.

Most people here are severely self-harming and complex. Some may have a forensic history (which means they hurt others and may have a criminal record).

A lot of people here have some sort of Personality Disorder.

I was in an LSU for a year.

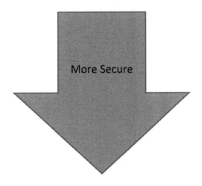

Medium Secure Unit

This is like a LSU except it is for people who have associated severe violent tendencies.

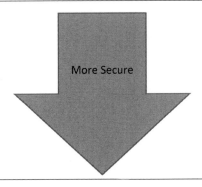

Forensic Unit

This is like a medium secure except it is for people with "forensic" histories, so they have a criminal record. This is the highest secure psychiatric unit there is for children and adolescents.

In adult services, there are high secure forensic units such as Broadmoor.

Whilst there is regular communication with a psychiatrist, electroshock therapy is no longer a mainstream treatment and is only suggested as a last resort. There are no bars over windows, they just open very little, an inch or two at the most. Sometimes the doors are locked. However in some units, they are not. Psychiatrists have pharmacists who have to check medication prescriptions to make sure that the doctors are not going over the legal doses, and Second Opinion Appointed Doctors are utilised after 3 months of being on a section to ensure that medication is used appropriately. Catatonia is not a frequent occurrence due to medical breakthroughs. Physical violence only really happens in more secure units if a person is particularly unwell.

Here is my story about such places. My story starts in the community, running away from my demons.

Just. Run.

That was my only thought. The blaring sirens became increasingly louder with each ragged breath. Their pounding seemed to be exactly like the pounding of my climbing heart rate. My lungs screamed for oxygen. Warmth seeped into my muscles whilst the burning of lactic acid infected every cell in my body. A stinging, itching sensation crept up my leg, seizing it, trapping it.

Just. Run.

Quick, quick. No time. Shaking my leg as though my life depended on it, I broke free of the nettles which remained determined on clinging to my lower body. I weaved my way through towers of trees, rapidly hurtling past blurs of buildings. I sped down the path, which was littered with pebbles, and dodged the phalanx of woodland beasts.

Just...

My footsteps slowed as I observed my surroundings. I'd stopped off at the local park area. Before me lay a river which was heavily polluted with plastic bags, empty cans, with a smooth coating of oil to top it off. The river was my brain, polluted with unwanted thoughts, tarnished with past memories, all glossed over with a fake smile. The thought of this made an investment in my tear bank, which (might I add) I had thought was exhausted; empty. Tears welled up, blurring my vision. My nose started to run. *Oh no you don't, hold back the river.*

A storm began to brew, as a shadow of despair and gloom descended over the lake. Thick clouds encompassed the indigo-stained sky. The overcast, saturated clouds started to rumble. As if almost ambivalent as to whether or not to cry. Dark grey undertones of clouds stood as a hindrance to the Sun, usurping full control of the sky. The clouds let go. They leaked.

Drips turned into trickles which turned into gushing of water like someone had emptied a bucket of water from in the clouds.

In a petty attempt to seek shelter, I concealed myself under a tree. The branches acted as a barrier between me and the exposed, open view of the sky.

Fear washed over me, down my back, slowly sinking like a dead weight in my stomach. My heart thumped as if it might just break free of my chest.

I could flee into the darkness. I could let the shadows welcome me back home, let them hijack the reins to my life. No, I'm tired of running. It's time to go back.

Chapter 2

Whacky Warehouse, Madman Manor

Madman Manor was my very first ward I was in. Originally I was here for suicidal thoughts. I only just turned 14 a few days prior, marking my 3rd year being depressed. I had an eating disorder, depression, anxiety and was freshly diagnosed as autistic. I was admitted for suicidal thoughts and a clear plan to end my life.

For people who first come into these units, they are very impressionable and want to know more about the different phenomena that occurs in hospital. I was no different. I became interested in people who were put on 1:1, the different types of secure and non-secure units there were and the different ways people used to self-harm. Like most young people, I had no idea such places existed and was fascinated by the different things that used to happen here. This is probably the first time I got sucked in to hospital and felt the almost-magnetic attraction to this kind of life.

There were a lot of agency staff members who didn't know a thing about mental health and could hardly speak English properly. There were very few permanent staff, maybe 1 per shift. It was shockingly bad and the ward manager was substandard and not a nice woman at all.

Whilst I was here, I had a big incident where I was moved from one of the quieter rooms to one next to the staff office where they could keep more of an eye on me.

Misunderstanding

When I was here, I had a misunderstanding, which I now realise to be part of Autism.

There was a Mauritian lady who liked me because I was Mauritian too and she used to keep rubbing my arm and I didn't like it. I wrote this in my journal and when staff found my journal, they thought it was a different type of touching so it was reported. That lady never even looked at me after that. She thought I was making an allegation against her but I didn't mean it that way. I just didn't want her to keep rubbing my arm and touching me!

"I can see the fairies!"

There was one girl who had bipolar and had 8 different admissions to hospital because she kept refusing her meds, leading her to become psychotic. She used to dance on tops of tables and say she was going to strip. She used to run in and out of rooms, saying how she could "see the fairies". She needed to be in a PICU (Psychiatric Intensive Care Unit), she was that unwell but they let her deteriorate instead. This happened when her mania went away, the depression came and she self-harmed severely, to the point of needing resuscitation. It was so sad to see her struggle and the staff increased her level of observations to 1:1. When she was well, she was quiet, polite and kind. She would go out of her way to help people and console the suicidal's. I felt like she had so much good in her, yet life treated her in this cruel way.

Eating Disorder Unit Programme

Whilst I was here, I had a time where I was really depressed and stopped eating for a bit. They said I had an eating disorder and put me on an eating programme for 3 weeks. These were the longest and most horrible 3 weeks of my life. I remember taking 2 hours to eat lunch and would be crying in the dining room. I had to wake up for 8am to have breakfast and would have 1 hour afterwards for supervision where I had to be sitting down, with minimal exercise, wasn't allowed to go to the toilet during this time. Breakfast was 2 pieces of toast with jam and butter and exactly 250 ml orange juice. Then snack would be at 10:30 and I would have supervision for 30 mins. Snack was 2 biscuits and 250 ml orange juice. The next snack was 3:00pm, dinner at 5:00pm and snack at 8:30pm. It was a lot and I hated being on this programme. It was so regimental and controlling. After the first 2 weeks, I stopped trying to fight it, after threats of being NG tube fed. Eventually my doctor said I didn't have an eating disorder, it was Autism...(I didn't know refusing to eat was a symptom of autism! Silly me!) This made me want to starve myself more, just to make a point to the doctor. Instead of doing this, I should have said, in hindsight: "Can you die of constipation? Because I am concerned how full of shit you are!"

I got close to other young people and thought they were going to be friends for life. Once I was discharged, I didn't speak to anyone from there because as soon as I was discharged, within 48 hours, I took a 50 tablet overdose which nearly killed me. I was put on IV Parvalex for a few days. As soon as I was physically fit, I was readmitted back into hospital, back to the same ward, but this time, on a section 2. I was put on 1:1, no bathroom privacy for 4 weeks. They even watched me while I was having a poo!

Chapter 3

Whacky Warehouse, Round the Bend (RTB)

I was here from September 2015-April 2016 the first time. I remember I was transferred there from the upstairs General Adolescent Unit but the consultant decided I needed a safer environment after my paranoia deteriorated and I presented with risk. The consultant for RTB, Dr Hayley Van Zwanenburg, was absolutely lovely. She was kind and understanding. Hands down, she was one of the best consultants I have ever had. She took the time to see what my interests were and, years later from RTB, still remembered me and that I liked Pretty Little Liars, the show.

The staff there who I really liked was Hazel, Sam, Maggie, Leonie, Krissy, Amie, Jainey, Neelam, Sarah, Laura, Sue, Kerry, Lynn. I had a really good bond with all those people.

At the time, I was really into Marvel and allocated a Marvel character for each staff member who worked on the ward and stuck it up on the wall but an unwell patient ripped it down during a psychotic episode.

There was one nurse who I despised secretly. She was like a round-faced, sassy, insolent Tinker Bell. She was an ideas generator but would rarely act upon these ideas.

Throughout my time on RTB, there were a variety of patients. One was a boy with schizophrenia and anger problems who was in my old unit but was transferred because of how badly he trashed his room. He smashed the bed in. There was a girl who used to be in a PICU (Psychiatric Intensive Care Unit) and she would have an incident every night. She was in hospital for about 2 years later on from that, she is now training to be a nurse! There was another girl who started to hear voices due to a troubled child hood, did drugs and attempted suicide, I think she was put into care after. She got pregnant at 17 I believe she is happy now, or so Facebook tells me. She was at my other unit too, but at the same time as me. There was a boy who had bipolar and used to get severely psychotic and manic to the point of hitting staff. He threatened to break my toes-how incredibly hard core! Eventually, it was decided his behaviour needed to be managed in a PICU (Psychiatric Intensive Care Unit). There was a high patient turnover, with a boy who I became very close to due to him saying I was his sister. He scared me at first because he was psychotic and shouting in what I later learnt to be Italian. We listened to Italian songs together and he would dance. He was quite the character but thought he was an alien. He used to go online and look at photos and say it was his planet. I remember how he loved his Parma ham and cheese- he would eat so much but never put any weight on due to his fast metabolism. After a few months, they transferred him to a PICU but when I spoke to him post-discharge, he still thought he was an alien. He was like a brother to me and it was heart breaking to see him go. Francesco, mate, you are a true legend and I hope you have an easy life.

There was another guy who kind of thought he was more unwell than he was. He used to say how unwell he was and that he needed to go to a more secure unit, despite his overall settled and calm temperament. I remember he had a panic attack right in front of me, spasming on the floor and they had to give him Diazepam but he was moving too much so was struggling to get the meds in his mouth. He was later moved to the GAU (General Adolescent Unit which is less secure) upstairs but he was hospitalised after he drank some substance from the cleaners' trolley. It was very scary. How could they discharge him after he did something so serious? I feel like staff thought of him as over-rating his illness so when he actually did something serious, they thought he downplayed it.

I recall another girl, Thalia who was stepped down from 10 months in a PICU (Psychiatric Intensive Care Unit) and I believe she was wrongly diagnosed with autism- I believe it now to be Borderline Personality Disorder. When she had flashbacks of her childhood trauma, she would get flashbacks and become aggressive. She also had an eating disorder and would secretly vomit in her bathroom. She told me but begged me not to tell the staff. At one point, she was Naso-gastric tube fed due to her eating disorder. This was when another girl was dragged to the clinic, kicking and screaming to get forced fed via Naso-Gastric tube. I think seeing this girl in such a state motivated Thalia's eating disorder to be just as bad. Years on, on Facebook, she left her supported living to live in Brazil and is now in another adult PICU. It is sad because I think it will take a long time until she is able to live in the real world and overcome her pervasive difficulties.

One person, in this admission who I think did the weirdest thing I have ever come across is a girl called Shakira who stuffed popcorn up her nose in order to be sent to hospital because she was bored and liked it in hospital. I wouldn't blame her, hospital is super boring!

A boy who was really aggressive came onto the ward and everyone tried to talk to him in sign language due to him being deaf. He was on 2:1 but due to his hearing impairment, he also had an interpreter with him all the time just to in case he wanted to communicate with anyone. I think this frustration of having 3 people with him every time was fuelling his aggression and he managed to break a window which was supported by 3 layers of supported glass. He was, consequently moved to a PICU because there were no beds available in any other deaf units. There was a girl on the ward who he had a crush on and so he tried to do inappropriate things to her which meant he had to be moved due to safeguarding.

There were a variety of different people I met on RTB. There was a schizophrenic boy who I had heard rumours about in regards to him damaging property and breaking an (what-was-thought-to-be) indestructible bed. He was very gentle and would fart a lot. It was gross. Everywhere he went, the stench would follow him. Ew.

Interestingly enough, I met someone who I believe had Multiple Personality Disorder. We used to talk a lot. One afternoon, she went into her room to go to the toilet. She was in there a while and when she came out, was banging on walls and doors, raising her voice at staff to let her out. Her whole body language changed, her facial expression, everything, but I couldn't put my finger on it. They let her in the garden and she was trying to abscond. Eventually she calmed down and sat in the corner. I tried talking to her and after half an hour of trying to get through to her, she said she was not Belinda, but "it". That was her name. "It". She said she didn't know who Belinda was and that she was an alien. After that, she fled to her room, to get away from us "strangers". I enquired about her behaviour to the staff who said she was just trying to get attention and was kicking off.

When she came back out, I asked her what had happened, to which she replied that she didn't remember and that she would have black outs a lot and had different personas inside her; an alien, a little girl, an old man... there were loads. After doing a mental health course later, I realised how it was actually Dissociative Identity Disorder or Multiple Personality Disorder.

If only staff hadn't dismissed her abnormal experiences, maybe, she would be in a better position for it...

At this time, I was in a bad place. I self-harmed requiring a trip to A&E and ended up on 1:1 for 4 weeks. This incident made me hallucinate worse than before. I remember I was hallucinating and was on a general hospital ward and the staff on my 2:1 (outside of RTB, I was on 2:1, 2 staff within arm's reach of me at all times) was sleeping and told me to go back to bed.

There was a physical health doctor was usually on-call by the name of Dr Ivan who didn't understand the concept of personal space and used to spend a lot of time with the girls on the ward. He was nice, just a little creepy.

One time, my friend on the ward told me one of the doctors was autistic. I asked the psychologist and she said it wasn't true at all and she got really angry with me. Afterwards, I had a meeting with the Medical Director who said that I was to tell no other patients which was fair enough but the psychologist didn't have to lie to me! They said that this doctor didn't want other people knowing about his diagnosis because it "may make the patients think differently of him". Although I respected his decision, I didn't agree with it because if I knew a doctor with lived experience of Autism, I would be more willing to engage with him because he would have a better understanding. If anything, it could have worked in his favour and mine! Despite my opinion, I respected his wishes.

This admission was one of which involved collusion with other patients. There was one girl who asked me for items to self-harm with. I gave her a box of raisins one time and she attempted to use this to self-harm with of which I had no idea. Later, she would ask me for stuff to use and at one point I was scared she was going to go to my room to get items. Eventually, I had to give the stuff I was using to a nurse so that this girl didn't get it. Another time, a girl who had bipolar disorder. When she was on a low, I remember we had a plan to break the fire alarm box to get the fire alarm to go off in order to get the doors to open and run out of the hospital. I didn't know what she wanted to do once she got out but I knew I was going to run in front of a car or lay on the road. In the end, we didn't go through with it and I am pleased I didn't because if we had made the fire alarm go off, we would have unsettled the patients in the whole hospital which wouldn't have been fair. I also shouldn't have teamed up with people to do this. It was really wrong of me.

I used to be the go to person on the ward to help the ward managers with posters and showing CQC visitors around. They knew they could count on me to help them with that kind of thing. I would give them a tour of the ward, starting from the front door and nursing station to the kitchen and door to the next ward.

At this time, my diagnosis was Autism Spectrum Disorder (Aspergers' Syndrome) and severe depression with psychotic symptoms. I remember they did a psychometric test which showed I scored high on the Borderline scale. When I asked the psychologist what it meant, she was very quick to say that it was inconclusive and meant nothing. If that was the case, why did she bother doing the assessment? It makes me think that if she had followed this up a bit more, maybe I could have had my BPD diagnosis and had got some help for it.

The environment was only slightly restrictive with TVs locked in see through cupboards and the kitchen was locked but we could go in there whenever we wanted (in reason). One time, they went on ward lock down and I thought it was because of me due to the fact that I went into the lounge and tried to rip something to utilise to self-harm and they locked the room for a week or 2 and I felt really bad because no patients were allowed in there, and it was all down to me! It was a horrible feeling.

When I started hearing voices, I remember staff saying how there was a patient who used to hear voices and they were really positive towards him, saying how he was a good person. One time, his voices told him that he was so good looking, he needed to go around naked because he was beautiful. Due to this, the medics put him on medication but he became depressed because he missed his voices because he thought they were good for him and he got incredibly lonely without his voices. This is more common than one might think. I know a lot of people who said that they wanted to keep their voices because they feel safer with them because they are like a friend. Sometimes the voices, even if they are not nice, are there for you, when real people aren't.

All in all, I built some really close bonds with staff, which I would later learn to become attachments which I found difficult to break. I was discharged from here to a residential.

Chapter 4:

Circle Road:

Circle Road was a residential children's home that I resided in for about 6 months in between hospital admissions. I was going to school and the residential was a really good place, better than most places in fact! The manager was so caring and when I went to hospital the second time since being placed in the residential, they fought to keep me and staff cried when I left I think the only thing that didn't work was me. My environment was fine. There were staff members who I got really close to and who helped me a lot when I was in crisis, such as the Fantastic Four (that is what I called them) and then there was K Gravy who fought tirelessly to ensure my place at Circle Road would not be lost after going into hospital. She was one of the best managers I have ever had.

The support network around me was perfect. It was just me, I wasn't ok. I needed more time (probably therapy) to explore the events that still haunted me. It was a place where I would struggle with self-harm and suicide for months- overdosing every few weeks and self-harming. In hindsight, I was struggling with secure attachments and didn't know how to express that in any other way and I guess I kind of wanted to go back into hospital so that I could see the staff from there. My secure attachments meant that I had severe trust issues and relationship problems to the point of being scared to trust, and when I did, I would become suicidal once they left. This added to my fear of abandonment because I my self-worth depleted when I thought nobody loved me.

The amalgamation of difficult feelings and such struggles became a cycle of self-harm and self-destructive behaviours, to the point where I did return to hospital and the same ward but little did I know how much had changed... It was no longer the same RTB I had grown to love and cherish dearly. It was no longer the same RTB with a fabulous, empathetic consultant.

Back To Hospital

Many staff had left and moved on-staff who had pinky promised they would never leave (the pinky promise is the most solemn of oaths and I believe the punishment for failing to adhere to it should be the death penalty but that is just my opinion, besides I digress). There was a new consultant and there was a new vibe that I got. I couldn't explain it at the time. It was probably a reflection of how Birmingham CAMHS had been changed to Forward Thinking Birmingham. There were even more agency staff than usual. Some staff had moved onto become ward manager of other wards. The ward was no longer the old RTB and they were moving buildings to a newly built one. The new building had heated floors and was a lot more modern. However with the modern-ness, came a more clinical setting, maybe too clinical. As we moved buildings, they said that they had to paint over the handprints.

What I mean by handprints is that when patients were discharged or transferred, they would get paint and put their handprints on the wall with their name and when they left. I did my hand print there as had many others. As we had to leave the old RTB, they told us that they had to paint over the handprints, which made me sad because all those people who had put their handprints there, thought they had left their mark in the ward and then now, they were being covered up. It was sad to leave all that behind.

Staff spoke to me about how they wanted RTB to be how it used to be and how they could tell it had gone downhill. I still think that they don't know how to change it.

CTO

After my 3rd admission, I was put on a community treatment order. The easiest way to explain it is a section in the community for which an individual has to abide by certain agreements or else will be recalled into hospital. For example, my terms of agreement was that I had to take my mental health medication or else I would be admitted back into hospital on a section. Due to the complex nature of my mental health, I stopped my medication and deteriorated, presenting with risk behaviours and was admitted back into a psychiatric unit under a section 3. This was my 4th admission.

Being placed under a CTO probably wasn't a good decision. You see, I have BPD and I had a complicated relationship with being in hospital. I would frequently stop taking my meds, get suicidal and psychotic and become emotionally dysregulated, meaning I had to go into hospital for my own safety. Most times, I would be admitted to hospital under a section 3. This is not usual.

Usually before someone goes into a CAMHS unit, (I can't talk about adult units) the young person needs to have a gateway assessment. If they consent to going into hospital, they are admitted as an "informal" patient. I never consented, thus needing a Mental Health Act assessment. Usually young people are admitted under this under a section 2 , which is for assessment. Section 3 is for treatment. My being admitted under a section 3 meant that the professionals involved in my care knew that I needed treatment quickly because they already knew what the problem and all I needed was a depot injection of meds in my system and then I would be out of crisis.

Depot is a type of IM, intra-muscular injection, where they give you a dose of medication usually in your bum cheek. I was forcefully given IMs on numerous occasions.

Now, coming back to why CTO wasn't a good decision. I had complex mental health problems. Whenever I was discharged from hospital, I would struggle in the community due to having to break attachments with staff in hospital and not being able to cope with this. For example, in hospital, young people are protected from harming themselves, they are told that they are cared for and given attention in a way that you don't get anywhere else. They save you from yourself, save you from taking your own life. Naturally, you would become close with these staff and I had attachment problems anyway so when I would leave hospital, I would become suicidal from the breaking of these attachments-that was how much it affected me.

Going into hospital was something I wanted because then I knew I was safe and I would get that validation from staff on the unit. Every time I was discharged, I would present with risk behaviours because then I knew I would go into hospital and people would tell me that they cared about me and would have my back. I got this emotional validation and attention only when I would be in hospital. Due to my BPD, I would think that any attention was good attention. I would stop my meds because then I knew I would become risky and unwell so then I would have to go back into hospital to receive that care and validation. Being on a CTO made that easier. Being on a CTO makes going into hospital a faster process. There is no waiting for weeks for beds because you are labelled as a priority so within a week of being risky, I would end up in hospital and I would be back to square 1 in terms of my recovery and it was just a never ending cycle of being discharged and then admitted again and after a 4 years of this, I broke the cycle by doing an intense course of 7 months of therapy. Although CTOs help some people, for example, people with psychosis or bipolar who are reliant on their medication to remain well, it needs to be reconsidered when it comes to people with neurotic illnesses and emotional problems.

Chapter 5:

Holidays in Hollywood

I came to Holidays in Hollywood (a physical health hospital) which led to my fifth admission to psychiatric hospital. I was actively suicidal and had made loads of attempts in the space of 1 night. I was restrained properly for the first time. I was put on 3:1 (3 staff being with me at all times) and was constantly trying to abscond from the general hospital, so much that the security guard had to stay with me. I was placed under section 3 within a few days. I was off my meds and was really struggling. I was depressed and wouldn't get out of bed, just crying all the time. It was at this time that the professionals around me had concluded that I was emotionally dysregulated due to my BPD.

I was given the news that I would be going to a PICU, a Psychiatric Intensive Care Unit. I was terrified! PICU was something people talked about on RTB ward and I had seen people be transferred to PICUs due to being really unwell and a great risk to themselves or other people. It was supposed to be a last resort due to the chaotic nature of the unit.

When I arrived, I tried to run to get away. I was so frightened when I got there. There was a boy spitting at staff and being restrained in the middle of the lounge, a girl hitting people with an NG tube in her nose and other young people I had met when I was on RTB unit and a girl who was following staff around poking them, a mere 2 inches away from them (I later found out she did this due to her attachment disorder).

At first, I hated it! I was crying every night.

I hated the environment. Patients were being restrained in front of me. It was too much of a sensory overload and most of the staff there couldn't speak good English (most staff were agency and most of agency were foreign or non-British).

I detested being stuck in such a secure place, to the point that I decided that I would fake it 'til I made it. I would pretend to be of euthermic equanimity in order to fool people to discharge me so that I could end my life. The medics thought I was taking my meds when actually I was secreting them. They had already given me the choice of taking my meds or having depot (injected medication against my will). All the people in PICU were too busy reacting to the incidents and behaviours of other young people to the point that I was missed out and people never suspected that I was actually not fine.

The doctor there (of whom I hated) said I didn't have BPD, despite me having it on my previous admissions' discharge papers. I am guessing that the reason why he thought this was because I wasn't histrionic or as dramatic as some of the other young people who had BPD.

I hated this place more than anything which is why I worked extra hard to move on from there so that I would be one step closer to my ultimate plan of being in the grave.

At Hartley, I decided I was going to secrete my medication and find a way to kill myself that would work but would try to play the system a bit to make people think I was ok so that I could have more opportunities to kill myself.

All I could think was that I would pretend I was ok, feign a calm equanimity, get discharged and kill myself. I had accumulated a large number of risk items in my room and it was every growing. My min was constantly thinking of things I could use to hurt myself. I would go to the on-site school there to fool the medics into thinking I was ok but I knew in my heart that I wasn't going to do my GCSEs because I would be dead by then.

I had no incidents in the PICU and the staff thought I was taking my medication so the medics decided I should be stepped down to an open unit, a General Adolescent Unit (GAU). Luckily there was a GAU onsite called Thorneycroft.

Chapter 6:

Holidays with Thompson

When I was moved upstairs into Thorneycroft, I had already gathered a large number of risk items. I was struggling to keep up my façade of being happy. I was becoming noticeable withdrawn. As soon as I got to Thorneycroft, I had set a date in 2 days' time to kill myself and had 3 different ways to execute this plan, and thus myself.

Eventually the day came; I planned to abscond, self-harmed severely to the point of needing restraint and then took an overdose. A staff member (who actually used to work on Mulberry) could see I was drowsy and knew I had taken an overdose and so called the ambulance. I was wheeled through the communal area in a wheel chair because I couldn't walk and then was observed for treatment. My heart rate was really high so I had to stay in the general hospital for a while in order to see it decrease. When I was fit to go back to Thorneycroft, I tried to run off again. I nearly made it but not quite. Staff restrained me in front of all the public. I was put on 1:1 observations where a staff member was with me 24 hours a day even in the toilet.

I grew bonds with staff this way. They spent time with me, got to know me a bit. It was also here that my paranoia got worse. I didn't sleep for 60 hours straight, I would only eat a bowl of cereal every couple of days because I thought this was the only way people wouldn't poison/contaminate my food. This led to me being NG Tube fed.

There was Preet (I would call her Preet stick), Ben, Lee and Bee. Ellesia and Michelle kept me safe when I had big incidents. Elaine the Pain, Rapunzel Gyanfi and Ellie Not-So-Swift were also there for me and were so kind to me.

One of the staff members, Ben, who I got on with, used to eat extremely hot food which would make him go to the toilet loads and be really...flatulent. He used to offer ghost chillies to people and say that they were actually just sun dried tomatoes. He played many pranks. When I was hallucinating, I entrusted him with this information and he was actually really caring. After I left, I found out he quit his job to continue being a plasterer. It was a shame because he was really good at supporting people.

There was a support worker who I really liked called Preet and I used to call her Preetstick (like Pritt stick) because she was the glue that was holding my sanity together. She used to call me gangsta ZeZe. She was bubbly and loud but approachable and kind. She would really cheer me up. When I was in the bathroom and she had to be in with me, I would be brushing my teeth and she would always tell me to "brush right at the back and get them molars the cheeky ones!"

Lee was there for me when I took an overdose and he was just so kind. He would have lengthy of conversations with me about how he didn't want me to die and he could see my potential. He believed in me. He was so altruistic, it was humbling. He would cheer me up and watched Fonejacker videos with me on the night before I left. It would be about pigeons being extracted from someone's bank account. For those 2 minutes of laughter, I forgot about the fact that I was going to a Psychiatric Intensive Care Unit and, for a moment, was just a normal girl laughing at a simple video. I would tell him how I needed to die and it was engraved in my heart to leave this world because I wasn't meant to be in it and how it hurt too much. He would argue with me over this. It was the kind of argument that made me feel loved.

Paddy Joe was a nurse who many people didn't like. He initially wanted to be an actor and went to drama school but ended up being a nurse...somehow. He says he shifted career prospects because he was just "too good" at being a nurse, but at the time I thought otherwise. He used to tell me stuff straight, so at times, I would hate him. He was there for me when I needed him to be. He did watch me have a depot injection and I hated him for it for a bit (a depot injection is when they inject anti-psychotic medication into my bum cheek) He told me that if I didn't come to the clinic to have my injection willingly, he would get staff to drag me up the corridor. I would act like I didn't like him but actually, I would find his presence to be comforting because of how much he knew about me. He was a nurse at Madhouse Manor and so he had seen me on my very first admission. He was the one who sent me to hospital when I took the overdose at Holidays in Hollywood. He was actually a really good nurse and I used to hate how he would psychoanalyse things and get it right. On my last morning, before I was transferred to PICU (Psychiatric Intensive Care Unit), he told me I would be OK as I was bawling my eyes out, terrified for my future. I wish I could tell him how well I am doing now...I want to show him that now I am ok and thank him for keeping me safe.

Whilst I was here, I did make some allegations during the time that I was delusional from lack of sleep. I regret this because I know that allegations can cost someone their job. I am sorry.

When I left, I was heartbroken because I had grown to trust in these staff members. Leaving made me lose hope. These people made me feel like I mattered and had a place in the world. Even at my worst moments of suicidality, they would understand me and tell me that they wanted me alive. They validated me and understood how much I wanted to die. When I was risky, they made me feel important.

When I was here, I created rules for staff to follow for when I was on 1:1 and then 2:1. Here is what I wrote:

- It is wholly unnecessary to open your fat gob every time you are observing the young person.
- Do not encourage the young person to be doing something every minute of every day. Allow them to sit down, think and check in with their emotions. If you prohibit this, it can be inferred that you are attempting to control their thoughts which leads to the perfectly reasonable conclusion that you are a control freak/telepathic tyrant.
- Don't call them "naughty" for being on 1:1. Being risky is not the same as "playing up".
- Forbidding young people to do certain activities because it is "too risky" is preposterous. The young person is already being monitored.
- Sleeping whilst on somebody's observations should give you the chance of being burned at the stake. These are people's lives in your hands. When you sleep, you are endangering people.
- Shouting among other staff members and therefore.

Chapter 7:

Cuckoo Kingdom

I was terrified of being here to start off with. This was my second PICU and at the time, I was very unwell. As I entered the doors, I self-harmed. I was paranoid and suicidal. A few days before hand, I was NG tube fed and IM'd (depot) in my bum cheek. I had just returned from a trip to hospital for serious self-harm and had not slept for 4 days due to paranoia. I was moved to the PICU against my will after the medics told me I was too risky for an open unit and needed a "more secure environment which could facilitate my long term behaviours". At the previous hospital, I felt as if the staff understood me really well. Very few people understood me as well as they did.

I remember on the way to the hospital, I was in secure transport with body guards and the radio was on. Due to not sleeping for 4 days, I was a bit delirious and thought the radio was talking to me which really frightened me.

At the PICU, I became attached to a few people whose names I later carved in my arm. It was Amy, Fidel, James and Ali. These people had a very firm understanding of my illness and my difficulties. I missed them so much after leaving. Even though I hadn't known them for long, I knew that they were good staff.

Fidel used to say I was like his little sister and every night, he would offer me my medication, which I would refuse. He knew I would refuse but would unfailingly offer me them every night because he knew they worked for me and that it would help me. He used to tell me that he would always care about me and just wanted me to be well because I had a lot of potential. He was so caring and understood about voices and that I needed help. He was so kind and this is something I will never forget. His compassion was genuine and came from a good place. Even though he would be really busy, he would always wave to me and talk to me to make sure I was ok. He was a really good man.

James (who I used to call Jimbo) was great too. He was my allocated nurse and as soon as I came, he said he would help me with my paranoia because he had helped a lot of people with my paranoia and would put things in place to ensure he could help me the best way he could. He was the one to put in my care plan about people taste-testing my food to reassure me it wasn't poisoned. He facilitated for me to sleep in communal areas because I was paranoid that people were going to hurt me in my sleep- he would work closely with the doctor to authorise this. As I got to know him, I found out he used to work in a medium secure where the majority of his patients had Borderline Personality Disorder. This made me think he could help me and that he understood because he knew a lot about borderlines. He got me to open up but every time I would spill something about my illness, I would get angry with myself for confiding in someone. He had a way of supporting me to get the information out of me. I simultaneously appreciated but resented this. I liked it because I knew he cared but resented it because I felt I had done something wrong by confiding in someone because my voices made me want to not tell people stuff. I used to say he had the mind-reading skills to pay the bills. We would have lengthy chats about my suicidality and how he was really worried about me because he knew how much I wanted to die and that he knew I was faking my presentation to get discharged and kill myself.

He used to say "I am not as green as the cabbage that I look" which apparently meant that although he looked gullible, he could see through my false appearance of seeming ok when he knew I really wasn't inside. I think it was just something he made up.

When I gave him my suicide note, I put on there: "Ding dong! The bitch is dead. Marvel at the borderlines. Bye Felicia." To which he asked me what language "Bye Felicia" was. I tried to explain what it meant.

Next up was Ella, a newly-qualified learning disability nurse and who was authentic and kind. She was down-to-earth and just lovely all around. I opened up to her about having Borderline Personality Disorder and she said that patients with BPD sometimes did struggle with psychosis. Whenever I would get overwhelmed with voices, she would sit with me and reassure me that they weren't real and that she was going to find a way to help me. Her reassurance was what I needed. Her altruism was refreshing as was her will to help. Most nurses, when they peak mid-career, they lose the reason why they went into nursing in the first place- to help people. Because she was fresh out of university, her intentions of nursing were well-founded and embedded into her practice. She would comfort me in times of dire distress.

Ali was the ward manager and probably one of the best ones at that! She introduced herself to me and I was going to help her to create a ward newsletter. I braided her hair and helped her with little odd jobs. She was lovely and very well-experienced. When I was told I was going to Low Secure unit, I told her that I had no idea what an LSU was and she looked online to help me to understand what types of units were out there which really helped to calm me down and reassure me that I would be ok. She always went the extra mile. She would come onto the ward at 7am at times. When I left, I tried to run off and was crying to her, saying that I didn't want to leave and she hugged and put our foreheads together, saying that I would be ok and that she knew I didn't want to leave. It broke my heart to leave there because at the end of my admission, the staff understood the nature of my illness and the complexities that came along with it.

Jimbo told me that the reason I like all of the above staff was because they were all learning disability nurses and apparently, patients with personality disorders take a liking to these kinds of nurses due to them being a bit "softer" and more compassion-focussed in their training.

With all these staff, I was scared to sustain the relationship and keep talking to them because I knew that Psychiatric Intensive Care Unit (PICU) was a short term placement and I would have to move on eventually and I knew it would hurt me a lot to get to know them and have to leave them via discharge or transfer. I used to tell them, "I don't want to talk to you because I know I will get attached and then get hurt when I leave you and I won't be able to deal with that because it will hurt too much".

All these staff used to understand that I struggled with trust and attachments. I would give them nasty letters saying I wanted to cut them off, when actually, I wanted to cut them off because I was scared of getting hurt if I trusted them.

I wish I could have stayed at this PICU because the staff understood me well however they knew I needed long term therapy which they couldn't offer me in a PICU because it was a short term placement for stabilisation, not for long term recovery. The doctor told me that she could let me stay and I would eventually stabilise but would soon relapse in the community and then come back into hospital and this cycle f hospital wouldn't stop unless I had therapy in a secure long term environment such as a Low Secure. If I didn't come to this unit, and if I didn't have my EUPD (Emotionally Unstable Personality Disorder) diagnosis, I wouldn't have been accepted into Low Secure, and if I hadn't been accepted into Low Secure, I probably wouldn't be alive today. The psychiatrist who referred me to the Low Secure was a really competent psychiatrist who listened and took me seriously. Without her, I would not have received the help that I got at the Low Secure.

The Deceit of a Snake:

There was a staff nurse called Sturdy who was the first nurse to sit down and talk to me when I was admitted. He didn't quite understand but was nice enough. He used to call me Jumbo because he knew I liked Jimbo. He held my hands when I was hearing voices.

One day, the patients on the ward and I tricked him into thinking there was a snake in the garden. We got the reception desk to tell him that the pet therapy service left a snake and were looking for it. We were told her was terrified of snakes, which made it even more funny! We said we could see something long and green moving about in the garden and got the rest of the staff to leave so that he was the only one who could go out. It was a foam snake that we made! His reaction was priceless and he jumped!!

Chapter 8:

No-View Hospital, Recovery Resort

When I first went there, I was terrified, sleep deprived and unwell. I hated it there for the first 2 months.

It was a nice welcome though. When I got there, I tried to abscond straightaway and they dragged me in safe holds to a room where they sat me down with the doctor. Later, I stayed in a room and they invited patients in one by one to talk to me and tell me a bit about themselves.

I was on Brenin Ward first but then was moved to Ebbw ward after 3 weeks. My paranoia made me fear falling asleep in case someone did something unspeakable to me which means I fought sleep for 5 days. I had my first IMs (intramuscular injections, for rapid tranquilisation) and floor restraints here. After my first IM, the Lorazepam knocked me out and I couldn't walk because of how strong it was. The more IMs I had, the more my body got used to it. I think I had about 10-12 IMs here, this wasn't a lot compared to some patients.

When I first got to Brenin, I was in anti-ligature clothing (which they called "Gucci gowns") a lot of the time and they used to do routine room searches every couple of days. When they did this, one of the staff members was looking through my notebook and saw an old suicide plan and confiscated my book. I felt really violated because that was my personal notebook!

Another time, I was being supervised with a pen with other people and although I was unwell, I was reading up a lot on quantum physics. I remember I was doing a quantum physics wave function equation of how to be discharged from hospital. Due to the different symbols I was using, the staff who was supervising my pen usage, handed over to the other staff that I was planning something dire because I was writing in a "different language" when actually it was just mathematical symbols!

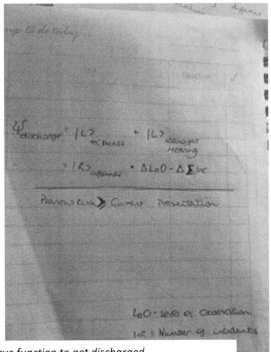

My wave function to get discharged

I used to sit outside the nursing office away from the other patients by myself. Very few staff tried to converse with me. Although I was actively suicidal, I was never as risky as some other patients.

These people knew me better than I knew myself. They were there for me at my darkest time and they stayed with me throughout the good and bad until I was ready to move.

I used to joke with staff that I needed a double vodka and coke to drown my sorrows, some people thought I was actually an alcoholic before coming into hospital. Truth is, I had (and have) never touched even a drop of alcohol. I haven't even had Listerine mouthwash (it actually has alcohol in it!). Whenever the staff would talk about going to the pub quiz in the local tavern after work, I used to tell them, "Please drink an extra vodka and coke for me to drown my sorrows!"

There was a doctor called Dr Ben. He was quite rude and abrupt. One time, a patient told him, "You tell me to take my meds once more and I will drop you quicker than you can drop your pants!" I was kneeling over with laughter, all the colour drained from his face and he hastily bumbled away.

Whilst I was here, I was very unwell. Just before I decided I wanted to recover, I became psychotic. I used to fight sleep for 5 days at a time because I thought people were going to die if I fell asleep. I also thought people were going to do things to me in my sleep.

I used to run into walls thinking they were portals. I had a delusion that I killed a baby and was a murderer because of a hallucination I kept seeing.

I punched a few staff. I don't know why I punched them, I can't remember, I was so out of it. I think I must have felt threatened in some way. I used to say and do things and then dissociate and not remember doing these things, as if I didn't have control. I remember I asked a staff member after my psychotic episodes what I was like when I was unwell. They said to me that one time when I was in a state, I just had a rapid tranquilization IM (intramuscular) injection and I had no bathroom privacy so I was having a wee and the staff member who was with me was standing in the bathroom and I said to her that I wanted to "strip because clothes were restricting." I have no recollection of this.

At one point, during my period of illness, I was in restraint for about 1 hour, maybe an hour and a half. Here at No View, they used to put people in floor restraints really quickly so I would be held on the ground against my will with 1 person on each arm, 1 on my legs and sometimes one on my head if there were enough staff. I think this was quite traumatic in some aspects, being held down for so long and not understanding why. I used to squirm a lot and attempt to wriggle my way out. It wasn't nice being on the floor, it was uncomfortable. I used to get bruises and carpet burns. Sometimes the floor would be really dirty too. Despite this, I was probably one of the more settled patients. There was one girl who would be in restraint for 2 or 3 times a day.

At this unit, all bathrooms were locked for patient safety which meant that sometimes, when the ward was busy or when the police had to come in to restrain patients (at which point I would dissociate due to being so unwell and overwhelmed with chaos, I would have (what I call) an "ill-timed urination". When the ward was not chaotic, it was so tedious so I would drink 4 litres of water a day out of boredom so that I would always need the toilet-it was just something to do but it worked against me because sometimes there would be no staff to open the bathroom for me because of all the restraints. It was far from ideal!

The Pen is Mightier than the Sword

The pen is mightier than the sword. This was probably one of the lessons from the Islamic Holy book, the Qur'an. I am a very relaxed Muslim so I wouldn't know the specifics. The reason why I bring this up is because this was a lesson I had to learn the hard way.

When I was in hospital, I discovered that I found writing down my worries quite helpful. Occasionally, nosy nurses would read my diary from time to time and usually they would confiscate it because of how negative my writing was. This was displeasing but not necessarily bothersome.

In these notebooks, I would write about my unfortunate dealings with staff, such as them being unprofessional. Eventually, they would find out what I wrote and speak to me at length about it and later hold a grudge against me.

Here are an example:

- Tonio who had a Tantrum and was tainted with (in)tolerance.

Tony was definitely of the Stark variety. Tonio was a nurse at my Low Secure unit and was (on approach) nurturing and nice but also slightly intruding but I didn't think anything of it. He used to talk to other patients in a way that was a bit out of line, saying that he was not going to accept their attention-seeking behaviour. One day, he made a joke in the communal area about one of his sexual experiences and I was taken aback by this. He also had a favourite patient who he would always support and not support other people as much. One time, I was having a bad day and took to externalising my emotions by taking it out on everyone else. At this point, I wrote him an articulate but harsh letter about his behaviour, telling him not to talk about his sexual experiences and demanding him to give the same level of support to everyone else, not just one patient. In response, he gave me a verbal diatribe (which I did not consent to!)Emmanuel where he addressed everything in the letter...but in a way I had not anticipated... He said that he was offended that I called him up on the sexual joke he made and said it wasn't true and he would never say anything as inappropriate as this, ever. He also said that I was being "homophobic" (which I am not, I am not sure about what kinds of people I like myself!) and said that because I was "Muslim [I] was different".

Woah! He did not just pull the "race" card? How does that even relate?

He followed on by saying that he remembers when I was really unwell and spoke to him about my psychotic experiences and he had to IM (intramuscular tranquilising injection) me because I was running into walls thinking they were portals.

That was low, he can't bring up experiences of my illness that I don't even remember! I was vulnerable, he can't use that against me!

Toni picked the wrong gal to mess with. Being the independent, strong woman I am, I reported this to staff and said he made racist comments towards me.

When he was next on, he said in front of the patients that he needed to have a chat to me because he "would not tolerate racist accusations". I spoke to him and he got an extra staff member with him so that it would be 2 people (him and staff) against 1 (me). He spoke to me at length about how he wouldn't let me get away with making false accusations about being racist because he isn't like that and has friends "of colour" himself. Everybody who is in denial about being a racist pulls the card about their "friends".

He said a lot of out of order things about how I never ask for support which is why nobody is willing to offer me any and I make it hard for staff to help me because I don't trust so easily.

If he knew more about me, he would understand why trusting is difficult for me.

He said my relationship with Emmanuel (the nurse who I nominated for an award- and he almost won!) was fractured.

He said that I have a "complex" that talking to my psychologist would solve everything and that he had a masters in CBT and my psychologist was only in training. In hindsight, he probably meant that he wanted me to open and widen my support network so that when my psychologist is not available, there are other people I can approach. Maybe, he didn't mean it like that and it was just a dig... who knows? Besides, I think it is good to only talk to my psychologist about my psychological issues. Speaking to nurses and support workers who may not have the same professional knowledge might not be what is best for me. Yes, good old Tony had a Masters in CBT but I was doing schema, not CBT and he might not know much about what psychological models to implement with different situations- that is the psychologists' job!

He also went to a new level of low saying that I "accused" my mother of doing exorcisms and she "didn't mean to do it"… he wasn't even there! He doesn't know half of the things I have been through. If this is how he thinks, he clearly doesn't want to help me. I know what happened and that is not something I misinterpreted. Other people know this.

Here is a poem:

There once was a man called Tony

Who sprouted a load of baloney

He pounced on my like prey

Called me a hater of the gay

I wish he was stomped on by a welsh pony

Birthday

I spent my 17th Birthday here. Before hand, I made an attempt on my life and tried to send funeral invited ready for my death on my birthday. My attempt didn't work due to staff vigilance but it did mean I was from that point on, nursed on 1:1 supervision in secluded areas. I didn't need to be on 1:1 all the time, just in quiet areas because that would be when I would be more at risk.

On my actual birthday, I asked for a buffet and the kitchen made me a unicorn cake with rainbow layers inside. We brought the cake down from the kitchen and just as they were about to cut the cake, the alarms went off and the staff ran away to see to it. I had a little cry because that was my big moment and everybody had scarpered to see to the incident. All the patients sat next to me to comfort me. After the alarm had gone off, the staff came back to cut the cake and it sooooo good. When the night staff came in, Matt, one of the good staff sauntered in, helped himself to some cake and said to nobody in particular, "Whose fucking birthday is it then?"

I said to him, bluntly, "Mine,"

"Aww, happy birthday Zee!" He came to give me a hug to which I tried to decline.

"I don't like being hugged or touched!"

He then replied, "Tough shit, Zee" and hugged me anyway!

Matt was great. When I was unwell and had a major incident, he said how it was really serious and when I was crying, he wiped my tears away and told me it would be ok. He was a brilliant, really competent staff member. He used to swear a lot, I remember but he was really good at communication. One time I thought he was Jesus when I wasn't sleeping for 5 days.

Copy Cat Behavioural Observation

When there are widespread episodes of self-harm in such as on the TV, a small percentage of people replicate this behaviour. It is an incredibly common phenomenon.

Why? Why would somebody want to mimic this type of action to their detriment?

In hospitals, it is called being a "copy-cat" which is an incredibly prejudiced term. It probably should have another name. In scientific psychology, it is known as the Werther Effect.

When I was in a Low Secure unit, there was a girl admitted on a Section 2 (for assessment, which is up to 28 days). She came in from home, with a drug problem. As she stayed, she observed many self-harm behaviours due to the chaotic nature of such a secure unit and how unwell patients can be. She started self -harming every day, something that she didn't do up until she arrived. She was discharged from the unit the day after she was admitted into general hospital for a self-harm incident. A week later, word got round that she was on a Section 3. She had ended up on a section which lasts up to 6 months due to her presentation which she had learnt off other people.

Another girl in another unit came in to hospital and learnt different behaviours from talking to people and ended up on 1:1 and in a PICU, 4 hours away from home. It was decided she was no longer safe/able to cope at her family home and was to move 2 and a half hours away.

A lot of people do this when they come into hospital. It is surprisingly common yet we still look down at people in disdain and condescension.

It doesn't happen just in hospital. It can happen in mild forms. You must have met someone in life who copies everything you do, much to your annoyance, someone who copies what you eat, drink, wear, do, everything.

It can happen in severe forms. Whenever film producers do storylines about suicide, it always provokes a reaction in the audience, so that they (the audience) in turn, ending up killing themselves. You must have heard of these incidents. Rates of suicide skyrocket when there is mention of someone doing this on the news or even on a TV show. Some people even imitated things that Jack the Ripper did.

So we have established that very few people like copy cats... but we are all copy cats, really, when you think about it.

When we are small infants, to learn, we copy what our parents say and do. We replicate to assimilate to society. It is part of human nature. I believe it goes back to evolution- we copy people to be accepted or else we risk exclusion. It is part of development. We copy-cat because we believe the outcomes of our actions are advantageous, we think this following observation of other people.

It is arguable that all behaviour is "learnt" behaviour but there are some ways I have self-harmed were completely original and thought of completely by myself. I can't decide if it is more detrimental to think up original ways to self-harm or if it being learnt is more detrimental. I think if someone were to self-harm and thought of it independently, it shows they have a more unstable mental state because they have thought deeply about it.

Some mental health clinical support workers argue that all behaviour is learnt behaviour, so everybody copies in some way.

Equality and Diversity in Medical Settings

In my Low Secure, I met some people with who had no appreciation for cultural diversity.

At this time, I wasn't on speaking terms with my family so it wasn't like I could talk to them to relay my worries so I bore the weight alone.

All the permanent staff were predominantly white and the agency nurses were mostly black. Any agency were mainly black. I was the only brown patient.

At one point, some of the other patients were watching a show called Citizen Khan about racial stereotypes of Muslim families. Eventually, the patients started extending their jokes to me and mocking how Muslims pray as well as talking to me in an Indian accent. Racist people disgust me. I can make jokes about my own culture, as I am entitled to that right due to being an ethnic minority. I used to make jokes about basic white girls but I have never been blatantly racist like they were. It is not like I called them "white devils"! Racism is a hate crime and it repulses me. I hated their actions. When I told staff about this, they took action and relocated a patient (the ringleader) to another ward. Yes, I would make jokes but never was I hateful to another.

On the subject of ethnic minorities, I went to a conference on recovery outcomes of which was revealed that young people and children of ethnic minorities are generally admitted into CAMHS services through other avenues of social care, usually by Youth Offending rather than the norm of going to the GP. This was interesting and made me reflect on the people who I had seen be admitted into hospital who were of an ethnic minority. Most of the boys who were BAME were there for psychosis and a few were violent (where they needed police to be involved). The boys who were of the same ethnic minority as me (South Asian) were there for drug-induced psychosis and some, autism. I met very few girls of the same ethnicity as me. It is interesting that this is the case but also shocking that this ethnic minority is missed when it comes to mental health support. It isn't that they don't have mental health problems, it is that they simply are not picked up by appropriate services.

Sick Boi

There was a staff member who I became really close to, Charlie. He was absolutely hilarious, used to make me laugh all the time. He was like the big brother I always wanted.

When he would eat, he used to look at the finger food in a funny way and go, "Ooooh, what's your name?!" before stuffing it in his face. He was brilliant.

People used to call him "Sick Boy" after a drug dealer in a movie that people thought looked like him. He had a bromance with another staff member called Connor Adams. They used to go to each other, "Alright, Di?" Sick Boy also taught me bits of Welsh. We used to always joke about the gym and getting "gains". We went to the gym a few times together and do body Pump classes, it was great.

Every time he used to come on shift, I would say," It's ya Boiiiii... SICK BOI!!!"

We had many inside jokes.

I punched him once when I was off my meds. If anything it brought us closer because of how guilty I felt about it. I started talking to him a bit more and eventually confided in him.

When I started doing well, other staff used to say to me how I didn't need to be in a Low Secure anymore. I tried to tell them how I was doing long term therapy and wanted to get this finished in a contained environment before moving on. Sick Boi was one of a few people who understood this and told me to take all the time I need. He understood that I was thinking of the bigger picture. Although I was self- harming less, I still needed to continue with therapy. You see, when someone stops self-harming, discharging them straightaway isn't the best decision because that young person can just as easily go back to those behaviours. As soon as a young person is ready to engage with therapy, it should be implemented. Long term therapy is the only way they are going to completely break that cycle of self -harm, through psychological intervention.

Sick Boy used to understand this. I think I would want him at my wedding, as the big brother I always wanted. The love I have for him is unconditional and I know that although I don't talk to him much, he will always be there for me.

Joe and Jodi Show

There were 2 shift patterns at No View. There was one who would work on Mondays, Tuesdays, Saturdays and Sundays and another who would work on Wednesdays, Thursdays and Fridays. They would alternate days like this.

My favourite shift was with Joe and Jodi. They used to have banter and Jodi would rip into Joe. She used to rip into Nathan as well, saying how his hair looked gross and he needed to lose weight. It wasn't in a malicious way though, it was hilarious. Charlie, Connor and Rachel Taylor used to be on this shift. It was great and they were my favourite staff members, I loved them together. I felt loved and appreciated when I was with them. Sometimes I wish I could go back to this because of how safe and secure I felt.

No View Raves

For a week, every night, there used to be faulty fire alarms which would go off every night at around 4am. The night staff used to call this No View Raves. They used to dance as if they were in a Rave. It was quite funny.

Attachments

It was at No View that people started to understand that people leaving was a trigger for me. When staff members used to leave, I used to find it really difficult.

There was 1 staff member who I used to be really close to, Craig. He moved to the other ward because he started a relationship with another staff member on the ward. He eventually left following some false allegations. I found it really difficult when he left. When Phoebe, one of my closer friends on the ward, left to go to adults' mental health systems, I was crying every day for weeks, same with the OT who left. Staff here understood that I would find it really difficult to trust and that when I did, I would relapse when staff would leave. In hospitals and care in general, there is a high staff turnover which doesn't help the situation anyway. When I did my long term therapy, my psychologist and I explored this and I came to the lesson I learned with her that "every relationship has a purpose,"

Other Low Secures:

Whilst I was at No View, I befriended a girl of whom we used to do yoga together every night. We had our inside jokes about autism. She had acquired brain injury which changed her personality (giving her personality disorder, otherwise called Organic Personality Disorder) and gave her learning disabilities too. She was lovely and I wish I could talk to her now. She had the same humour as me. Due to her learning disabilities, the medics sent her to a Learning Disability Low Secure. Her condition meant that she would present with risk behaviours in order to get put in restraint. I think she liked the feeling of restraint and being held tightly. The medics bought her a special tight vest to mimic the same feeling of security and tightness. It was quite an anomaly but I think it was because of her complex nature. She had some traumatic events happen to her, which she spoke to me about once. She went through so much, it isn't surprising that she wanted to feel safe and secure.

Once I rang her up and she was talking about her unit where there was a girl who was kept in seclusion for 2 years and the girl's parents went to court to get her to come out of seclusion because it was against human rights. When that girl was taken out of seclusion, she was very violent and displayed severe aggression. It was scary to think how dangerous this would have been.

There is another example of a hospital where it had a poor standard of care and a group of patients broke into the medication cabinet and one girl overdosed whilst another girl made a serious attempt on her life whilst it was all going on and ended up in a coma. The girl who ended up in a coma ended up in the same Low Secure as me and turned 18 quite swiftly. I remember she was speaking on the phone to her social worker, begging them to send her to an adult Locked Rehab (which has less security) instead of an Adults Low Secure (where it is harder to get discharged and it is possible to stay there for a number of years). In the end, her risk was deemed too high due to her past incidents and she went to an Adults Low Secure where she for a few years. This was also very saddening because she had so much potential and was very intellectual and witty. Mental illness nearly killed her. Once they sent her to the Adult Low Secure, I think she may have been more inclined to give in to her self-harming and suicidal ways. Going to adult Low Secure made her give up on the mere notion of recovery. It is heart-wrenching to know how much she has been through. It also made me realise how real the possibility of someone losing their life to suicide is.

Behaviour vs Mental Health

I really miss the girl who used to do yoga with me. I wish I knew what happened to her. She had been on 1:1 for about a year and was very complex. Staff used to say that her self-harm was mostly behavioural and so they would be dismissive of her struggles.

In hospital, health professionals identifies self-harm actions as either "behaviour" or "mental health" When it is mental health, it usually connotes more severity and people are a lot more responsive because they realise that people are actually mentally unwell and need to be in hospital. When it is "behaviour" professionals usually dismiss this behaviour and won't take the individual so seriously because they believe that the patient/service user did this action with specific intent, usually for attention, but in the absence of mental health. From what I have observed in hospital, these patients/service users have autism or a learning difficulty.

I never used to understand it, because there is always a reason for a behaviour and surely this should be seen to, and the persons' needs met rather than being prejudiced against this?

All behaviour is for a reason whether that be for attention or to illicit a response.

The Lucy Who Took Lucy Who Turned Into Lucifer

One of the many pleasurable individuals I came across was Lucy Donnybrook of whom I watched work her way up to one of the most secure units in the UK.

She came into a PICU for Drug Induced Psychosis and self-harm but she stayed for Personality Disorder.

She was at that unit for a year before being transferred to a Low Secure Unit where she stayed for another year, before moving to a Medium Secure Assessment Unit.

However, it felt longer than a year. It was a year of anguish, struggle and violence. I don't say this light-heartedly: Lucy's case was a prevalently dire one because when her illness took over, that was it.

She would lash out, in a very extreme manner. If she were to be restrained from harming herself, she would have externalised violent tendencies. This would include; scratching people's eyes, biting them (to the point, people had to have tetanus injections), kicking them in the ribs (and hence breaking them), punching staff (to the point of broken noses). Her attitude towards people would go much further than simply physical assaults-verbally attacking people, calling people with ED's fat and telling suicidal people that they should go die.

She hurt a lot of people in very serious ways. Many people were scared of her. She was on 3:1 with 2 extra support staff allocated to her in case she had an incident (technically 5:1). She would have to be subjected to an especially strong type of sedation called Accuphase which would have to be administered as an intra-muscular injection twice in order for it to have an effect. When it did have effect, she would be knocked out for at least 3 days. Accuphase is used sparingly, reserved only for the most chaotic of presentations.

Despite, the severity of the people whose lives she endangered, she was actually a very pleasant young lady with a good sense of humour (when she was OK, that is). This was just how her mental disorder manifested itself.

Many people thought she was just a bad person. It could be right, it could be wrong. It just goes to show that anyone can be affected with mental illness, regardless of what is in your heart.

Santa's Sweets

Today, a group of us went on Section 17 leave, got all geared and dolled up, got excited… to go see a light being switched on.

That's right, people, people in today's society have nothing better to do with their lives than to watch street lights being switched on during the Christmas period. It was nothing special, just a couple of half-hearted outlines of a Santa on a sleigh with a pathetic string of fairy lights. I only went out as an opportunity to get off the ward, an opportunity I grabbed with both hands (much to my dismay).

Eventually, after what felt like a lifetime, the lights came on and a fake Santa sat on a fake sleigh, being driven by a Santa's fake assistant in some random dinosaur costume. I watched with a glazed, emotionless expression as they passed, when suddenly I had an idea…

With a renewed sense of purpose, I walked up to the sleigh and called out to the dinosaur. By this time, Santa was going off to talk to some toddlers, being the little weirdo he is.

"Yo, mate!" I exclaimed.

I was met with a slightly apprehensive, "Yes?"

"We're from the psych ward at the top of the hill, it would really make our day if you would be kind enough as to give us some sweets. We don't get out much, see." It took every ounce of self-discipline not to burst out in laughter.

He pointed to Santa.

So I went to Santa.

"Hi, we're from the mental hospital up the road, it would be great if you could give us some sweets. We don't get fed very often."

"I'm so sorry but all the sweets are gone," he said.

Accepting this response, I walked away with a heavy heart.

Little did I know what a conniving manipulator Santa was!

It wasn't until I looked back that I discovered that Santa was giving sweets out to little children… "Sweets" he said he didn't have: he lied to me. That little

BUM! He may have thought I was joking but even if he did think that, it was awfully petty of him.

We deserve sweets more than little children. Those children are loved and cared for more than enough. We are vulnerable young people, many of us have suffered traumatic experiences. We needed them more.

In hindsight, I should have given him a tap. On the back. With a chainsaw.

However, if I had done so, it would run the chance that I would be detained on my Section 3 longer than necessary.

Utterly disappointed, with a depleted faith in the kindness of humanity, I returned to the Low Secure Unit.

Fang Shen Baa: Religion of Tea

There was a staff member called Maverick, who had got me to open up about my struggles a little bit and we had a lot of banter. I did, however stop talking to him ever since the day he left the whole ward unattended so he could go for a cigarette. I thought it was a bit reckless so stopped talking to him but in hindsight (and with the spirit of religion) I should have forgiven him. He showed me the light to Fang Shen Baa.

I am a co-founder of a completely original religion, which although is widely practised and sworn by millions, it is an unofficial faith. People of any background will sit together, regardless of ethnicity, sexuality, race or age...It is the glue which binds humanity together; tea.

Whether it is herbal, decaffeinated or maybe just iced, there is no discrimination. People from all over the world will unite (on a daily basis, might I add) to bond over a sanctimonious cup of tea and a chat. The Earth dying? Have a cup of tea. World War III starting? Have a cup of tea. Aliens swarming the planet, have a cup of tea. It is a world-wide, timeless solution.

Many people are (unbeknown to them) a follower of Fang Shen Baa, a religion I co-founded, revolving around tea being the purpose of life.

The Holy Scriptures are in a heavily bolted fault deep in my Mind Palace, called the Book of Nigel. Its main message is that you should always think of the cup of tea being half-full, never half-empty, we have to "keep it pozzy" (actual verse).

Derek, the Almighty Teabag of Life, is the monotheistic deity of whose message is to love and drink tea. He will forgive anyone as long as they refrain from committing the Major Sins:

1. Drinking coffee.
2. Putting milk in before the hot water.
3. Leaving hot tea until it gets cold, then drinking tea.

Minor sins include:

1. Not offering visitors tea.
2. Not praying (praying rituals consist simply of drinking tea)

365 days a year, is the Festival of Clive, in which one would celebrate and- guess what..? Drink tea.

Pervy Pablo the Perverted Pirate Pigeon is the devil. You just can't trust pigeons, they are sky rats.

Some prayers we have are as follows:

"Give tea to thy neighbour"

"Have tea and be kind"

"Tea will guide you to the right path"

...Yes, I can now see how I got sectioned.

A story I wrote when I was approaching fully-fledged psychosis:

It had all changed by the time I returned home.

Everything started when my work colleague, Peter Pan needed me to stay to participate in the Great Enchanted War. I fought my way through Sirens and won over the blasted she-devils. After a tedious, perfunctory battle, the Neverland Realm remained strong and protected. I wanted a battle which would ensure my legacy and martyrdom, not a half-hearted bar fight between 2 water nymphs. I needed an honest quest with a grand war. I needed an exhilarating, adrenaline-pumping challenge. I am allergic to boredom, it breeds eternal misery. I need to be mentally challenged in a similar way to how a baby instinctively craves his mother's milk.

I swiftly opened up a portal to the next universe; Asgard. The first thing that hit me was the purely putrid, foul-smelling stench that seemed to infect every cell in my body. It stunk, vile enough as if a God...

"Felicity! Felicity! Please would you do me a favour?" The stench grew stronger.

"What on earth is the matter, Odinson?"

"I appear to be suffering with severe bowel distress." I have been afflicted with great pain and rock-hard stools." Thor explained, his face contort with agony. "Please contact an apothecary, the Asgardians can't know their King is blocked up."

His request was seen to, however, I did "accidentally" put the whole conversation on the Avengers Group Chat...

Next, I needed to see my boyfriend, Spider Man. Peter and I went to a restaurant after the Battle of New York. As I was biting into my pizza (the Avengers got shawarma), I felt something shiny and cold. Picking it out of my mouth, I realised it was a ring...

"Will you marry me?"

Shocked, but pleasantly surprised, I slid it down my finger and hugged him, his arms wrapping around me in a safe embrace; it was meant to be. Warmth radiated through my solar plexus.

My final destination was homebound. As soon as my foot stepped on Narnian soil, I felt suspicion in every fibre of my being. The sky consisted of mackerel clouds, crimson and amber-tinted as if tainted with blood. Ominous clouds threatened rain. The wind howled like a desolate, frightened infant. From under the rocks, grew anthropoid-like creatures... aliens.

It really had changed.

Christmas

This Christmas, a surprise was scheduled. Donkeys and reindeer came in a barn in the car park. We petted and fed them.

Last year, I held the cousin of Rocket Raccoon from Marvel's Guardians of the Galaxy, as well as a skunk. I ran with Shetland ponies in a locked garden. This was all in a PICU, psychiatric intensive care unit. I remember we had to go to the secure garden.

For the Christmas Show, we did the Craziest Showman (loosely based off the Greatest Showman). I wrote the script and played with the lyrics to make it fit in with the theme of mental health. It was incredibly stressful and, despite it having a positive outcome, I would very much like to never do that again. Staff told me, "Every second you're not in education, you have to be doing work for the Show." No pressure, obviously.

Here is what some of the lyrics were from the first song:

"Patients and staff, this is the moment you've waited for

WOAH!

Doctors diagnosed me, no one can seem to find the cure.

WOAH!

My mental illness,

Is stealing my mind,

Trying to leave my negative thoughts behind,

Tryna fight it, it's coming for me,

Running 'atcha,

Tryna get off 1:1,

Don't care what's after,

Don't surrender even if you feel it taking over,

Obs are higher,

No freedom,

Home leave coming closer,

It's the doctor in the clinic doing the rota,

There's someone screaming in every room that's holding,

Hospital's all I know,

And I really just want to go,

Late handover taking all night,

My 1:1 checking if I'm alright,

My worst dream comes true,

Meds taking over you,

Oh, this is the craziest show!

It's something that you'd never want,

But it's something that you maybe need,

Especially if you're detained on a section 2,

Or even worse, a section 3."

Christmas is about presence not presents. This goes for any cultural or religious celebration, even if it is just your birthday. When I say this, I mean that it is supposed to be about family connections and making the most of the time one has with people they care about. It isn't supposed to be about the regular commercialised idea of Christmas with spending ridiculous amounts of money on family to the point of bankruptcy. It is not about competing with other people about how many presents you got.

Since I was younger, I have celebrated the Islamic festival of Eid twice a year, instead of Christmas. We would go to my Daddima's house and my uncles, aunties and cousins would congregate to share traditional foods, wearing celebratory clothing and giving out presents. In hindsight, presents are not that important. It is the love and compassion for each other that is important. The only thing I cared about was the gifts I got.

This is why it was a shock when I went into hospital and did Christmas, it made me realise how you can have expensive presents, but if you don't feel the love and support of people around, it isn't a celebration. In fact, it breeds eternal misery.

The End of No View

Left my Low Secure Unit for an Open unit today. 12 staff waved me off in the car park at 8:15 in the morning. They ranged from cleaners to psychologist,

OT's, nurses, support workers, admin staff, even the chefs who I used to get on with.

I felt loved. There were 6 people either side of the car.

When I came to the Low Secure, I thought nobody would care at all if I just killed myself. I hated everyone there and thought that the feeling was mutual. They meant nothing to me.

I never would have thought they would have such an impact on me and that I would come to love them. It took months for me to trust them and get to know them, but they were patient, more patient than they had ever been in any other unit.

Leaving, I felt deeply cared for. Feeling that I meant something to someone else gave me overwhelming happiness and contentment. I do matter. They will always think of me fondly and care about me. That isn't something I could get anywhere else in the world. They saw me at one of my darkest time and they nursed me to recovery. I wasn't completely recovered but I knew I was on the path to it. I was on the road to recovery and it was all due to their help. They took the time to get to know me and supported me throughout each blip.

It was here, at No View, where I had my turning point. I decided after my big suicide attempt here that I needed to start getting better. There was no way the people around me were going to let me kill myself, no matter how much I wanted to go. There was no point trying to fight the system. I needed to just try recovery.

And I did it. I worked so hard to open my can of worms and then neatly order them back into a better can, one that was more manageable. It was here that I was given the chance at therapy that I so desperately needed. I was successful in learning how to want to live.

My time was over. I could no longer live the No View Dream. I had outgrown them and there was now nothing more they could do for me now, through no fault of their own. There is and always will be a special place in my heart for these people. Rachel, Joe Smith, Jodie, Nathan, Charlie, Craig and Amy. I will never stop caring for them because of how much they have done for me. They saved me from myself. They helped me to find my will to live and I wish for them to be paid in glory.

Chapter 9:

Porangi Clinic, Heathens

After No View, I decided to take charge of my care and ensured I went to step down before being discharged to the community. This step down was supposed to help the transition between hospital and the community due to how long I had been in hospital for (4 years). Hence why, I went to a General Adolescent Unit in Birmingham, in my home town. The original plan was to send me to an ASD residential school however when I looked at places, I realised I wasn't autistic enough for those kinds of places and it would take about 6 months to get to be referred there. Even if I did go there, they might not have accepted me from such an extremely restrictive environment such as a Low Secure. In the end, I decided to be stepped down to an open unit and then go to Supported Living instead because mental health was my main problem and an autistic residential might be more skilled in dealing with autism.

So I came to Porangi Clinic.

There were very few staff I liked. There was Eloise who was funny and was always there for me. She couldn't handle chilli hot foods- she even thought toothpaste was too spicy! There was Jess, who I interviewed to get the job as a clinical support worker and who was a basic white girl because she had a fiat 500 (which apparently all basic white girls had). She was absolutely lovely but didn't say bye to me before leaving. Then there was Jimbo who was hilarious. Whenever I had my meds and fybogel, I used to mix the sachet with water and he made up a song:

#She likes to mix it, mix it,

#She likes to mix it, mix it

#She likes to mix it, She likes to MIX IT!

He used to pass wind when patients were crying in order to make them laugh. He was besties with this man called Neb, who spoke too much and although he had the best of intentions, he was just too lively and too much as a person, in the way of asking questions. There was Kirsty who used to work pretty much every day. She was on another ward but used to pick up loads of overtime and so that is how I came to know her. She was so good at what she did. If she wanted to, she could have been a doctor, she was so competent and clever. She really understood the complexity of my mental health and personal situation, she was fabulous!

The MDT at Porangi Clinic were great! There was Dr P who was hilarious. We became really close and we were quite the duo, always laughing together. She used to tell me how she used to go to the gym once a year. She went 3 years in a row once and 1 month, she went nearly every day but then left it for another year! She cracked me up! We had an inside joke that when I got discharged, she could come to my party and we could collect all the items which are usually contraband in hospital and put it in my flat as a celebration; machetes, rifles, knives, rope, EVERYTHING! We had a wicked sense of humour together. She even took me out for cake on my birthday! We went to a conference together where I spoke about recovery outcomes at the beginning of my co-production journey.

Next, there was Stocksie (that was what Dr P used to call her) and she worked with my social worker to secure me a bed at a supported living. She came with me to view places. She was very efficient and worked very hard as a Complex Discharge Co-ordinator (the only person I had come across in all my hospitals with this job title!) She was quite the character and used to go out with Dr P to view placements and would always find a way to get to a coffee shop to do a bit of "skiving" and have cake dates-we called it "community integration". She used to have quite expensive taste- one time, I went to an NHS awards ceremony with her and she said she rang up the taxi company that was taking us to ensure a Mercedes was booked so that we could turn up in style!

Then there was Ellie who taught me how to take the bus and now I use it every day. She was amazing! Funny, slightly reserved but still an extremely hard worker. She would stay until 6 or 7pm to do work.

The ward manager, Cathmandu, was also really competent and hard working. We worked quite closely together when I had a blip and she supported me through it. There was good old Paula as well who spoke with me to think about how to improve the service and we have started some co-production work.

I had my 18th Birthday party at Porangi Clinic. Ellie, Stocksie, Catmandu and Dr P came to have some cake and it was lovely of them, especially since Dr P came on her day off.

Throughout my time at Porangi Clinic, I went to the school on-site where I was usually one of the only students in the class. I came to the school in January when I was admitted and I was clear in telling them that I wanted to sit my GCSEs in May and do iGCSEs because I thought my Education team was going to sort this out for me. The education team didn't sort it until it was too late so James Brindley took me on and got me through what was supposed to be a 2 year course, in less than 6 months. The teachers were so lovely! They believed in me and at first, thought I might not be able to do it but they trusted I would work hard and I did, proving to them that I would not squander this opportunity. There was Alice, Sammy-Jo, Suzy and Linda, these people were my favourite. Linda gave me positive affirmation cards which told me to believe in myself and that I could do anything I put my mind to. She also did mindfulness with me during the exam period. Sammy-Jo used to give me this mantra during exams: "I can do this, I've got this, I am a boss." I will smash this exam. Alice, got me through so much content and was just all round pleasant and supportive of me. It was a great school and I couldn't praise them more highly. I am now the James Brindley Alumni and will return to talk about how well I am doing now. I also had prom here. It was a magical night and the best prom I could ever have imagined. I felt so loved and appreciated.

Because Porangi Clinic was an open unit, my mum thought that (due to it being less restrictive than No View), you were allowed anything and everything. So she brought knives onto the psychiatric unit. Let me tell you, that did not go down well. *FACEPALM* She did mean well and she didn't realise so lets give her that.

Area 51

On Facebook, there are loads of people saying how they are going to storm Area 51.

~~Let's storm Area 51, they can't stop us all.~~

Let's storm CAMHS, they can't section us all.

Pengalengous

The ICT teacher at the hospital school is retiring this year and it is only this year that she has had the lightbulb name for a "tag" to make her seem "hip" and "cool". Her name is Pat and her tag name is p@.

P... then ...@ .P@. Pat

She was so pleased with herself. She is simply brilliant.

At the Porangi Clinic performance of the Craziest Showman, one of her lines was to say, "You look well peng!" She is extremely well-composed and a tad posh so when she said that, nobody could stop laughing. Later, she told me she searched up what "peng" was online since she just didn't know why people found it funny. She also reported that she discovered the antonym for "peng" which was "leng" which apparently defines as "ugly". She was absolutely intrigued by this, wanting to research the background of this new language. Hilarious!

When I was at Porangi Clinic, I had only a couple of blips. My only one resulted in self-harm and verbally abusive letters to staff. I did, however, use my skills that I learnt in Psychology at No View and got through it with Dr P and the ward manager. It made me realise how far I had come.

Miscellaneous Pride

Today I have completed all my GCSEs. I had 19 exams in the space of about 5 weeks. It has been tough. I had to fit my GCSE course in the space of less than 6 months because my last hospital had a substandard education provider which only did Maths and English which had to be the welsh exam board- don't get me wrong, I made the most of it and went to each session however I was very limited in terms of resources, textbooks and qualified teachers. Whilst I was at this hospital, I made the decision to take iGCSEs, international GCSEs that I could teach myself and learn independently, however I didn't know how difficult it was going to be because iGCSEs have harder content- for example the Maths iGCSE includes matrices, a Further Maths A level topic- not just Maths A level, *FURTHER* Maths A Level. When I came to this hospital, the teachers supported me to do iGCSEs for all subjects.

- The English iGCSE had really strange and random books which I had to analyse, stuff which normal students wouldn't analyse at GCSE- Mansfield Park, A View from the Bridge and then obviously Macbeth (everyone does that).
- I have already touched on Maths iGCSE
- I did a lot for my Physics iGCSE and got a lot of teaching about this.
- Chemistry iGCSE was mainly self-study which was really difficult.
- Biology iGCSE was half-taught, half self-study.

For the Sciences, the textbook didn't follow the spec so I had to use the internet mostly for the content.

- Computer Science iGCSE- I have never done this before and my teacher didn't know any computer science, only ICT. I didn't learn the programming because we didn't have enough time and the teacher didn't know it.
- Despite all this, I still completed 7 GCSEs in less than 6 months.

My new college has a mental health team there.

Chapter 10:

I have been to 2 acute wards, 2 Psychiatric Intensive Care Units and a Low Secure, I have been moved across the country- from Staffordshire to Sheffield, to South Wales (where I was in a secure unit for a year) and then back to Birmingham... and I still have completed my GCSEs, against the odds. I went from being on 2:1, making serious attempts on my life in a secure unit, being psychotic, struggling with Emotionally Unstable Personality Disorder... and now here I am; becoming a mental health ambassador with different organisations, being an Expert by Experience (as a job) with a university, being Research lead for a mental health service improvement group, being considered to be a young person advocate to inspect mental health inpatient services across the country, training junior doctors on how to communicate with adolescents and I am also the most well I have been for 7 years! Look at me now. I am immensely proud of myself (in a non-arrogant way). I have come a long way in my recovery and I still have a while to go.

I am discharged boiiiiiiii. I am no longer shackled by the chains of detention under section and released from institutionalisation

Things are really good for me. Pride is currently radiating off me. It's a good time to be alive.

Phase 2:

Miscellaneous

Resurrection

Chapter 11:

Mental Health Ambassador: Its role in my life.

Being a mental health ambassador means so much to me.

It gives me a chance to be part of something bigger than myself, giving me a much-needed sense of belonging. When I was younger, I never felt like I belonged anywhere, I wanted to matter and be important. I remember when I was younger, asking my mum, "Where is home?" She would reply, "You are home." But I didn't feel like it was home, I felt I didn't belong.

It all comes to validation. I wanted someone to validate me and prove my self-worth to me. I know now that the best way to do this is to self-validate or not rely on validation from other people as much. Being an Expert by Experience or a mental health ambassador gives me that automatic validation by the fact alone that people turn up to talk to me. They are genuinely interested in what I have to say.

The group that I am with, Think 4 Brum, is an Expert by Experience group of young people and I get a lot of support from them. It is refreshing to be in the same room as people who are so passionate about mental health, just like me.

This is the same for the Institute of Mental Health's Youth Advisory Group at the University of Birmingham. I advise on research proposals linked to youth mental health. It is incredibly humbling to think that advising on this research could help save other young people from poor health.

It is also about giving back to the community and thanking the world for everything it has done for me. The mental health system has done so much for me and I need to repay them by offering my services.

This kind of work helps to appease my suicidality cycle because when I get to the point of suicidality and feel I can no longer go on I think that even if I can't live for myself, I will live for others instead. Instead of throwing my life away, I can make use of it for the benefit of others; by helping people. I will devote my life to other people. I will try to show love to them, even if I hate myself.

There are so many other people suffering out there in the world and they want to live. I don't, but they do. Why should I throw away something that they want if it could save their life? My aim is to kill myself, I don't need to hurt other people in the process.

Sometimes I think that I should donate my body to science, allow people to cut me and take my organs. I would die in the process but at least I could have helped people. This way, I would get what I want and they would get what they want too which would have been ideal to me previously.

Now I have a greater sense of value my life, I know that I am worth more than this and I have a whole life I don't want to waste.

Doing mental health ambassador work has boosted my self confidence in this way because it has taught me that I can make big changes to the world around me and can contribute to society that still preserves my dignity and self-respect. It has revealed some self-truths that I can do anything I can put my life to and my determination (which could be perceived as stubbornness) is a motivator and driver. Instead of using this drive for maladaptive reasons, I can apply this to the improvement of society. My family would always say I was stubborn and (although I didn't realise this at the time), this is an incredibly positive trait, in fact, maybe even sought-after for some people!

I think it is with this type of work, I have found purpose. Everyone finds their purpose eventually, and I found it after 4 years in psychiatric units. I am part of something bigger than myself.

It also makes me think that I am making the most of my situation. Yes, it was horrible to have been institutionalised for so many years and to have gone through the ordeal I have been through, but if I hadn't experienced any of that, I wouldn't be where I am today- giving lectures and sharing my story. Yes, I have been IMd (types of injections for rapid tranquilisation or to inject anit-psychotics into me), restrained to the floor and I have been through so much emotional pain but if I wouldn't be the strong young woman I am today without any of that. As much as it is hard to admit, I am happy that I went through all of that, survived it, because now I am happy, strong, healthy and resilient. I have experienced a lot in life at such a young age, some things of which most young people my age have never been through at all! It has made me a better, kinder person.

After all, who else will know what a good mental health service is like than the people who are experiencing it themselves?

Chapter 12:

The Miscellaneous Mentally Ill

I met a variety of different characters throughout my time in hospital. Some of them, I wonder if they are even still alive. On social media, there are increasing occurrences of mental health hospitals shutting down after patients manage to end their lives there. It is frightening to think that people are struggling so much and no professionals can see that. I will tell you someone who does see that- fellow patients. Nobody understands the struggles more clearly than other patients. Here are some stories about some patients who I wonder about from time to time.

One boy used to be really rude and was almost obsessed with fricklefrackle. Everything was an innuendo to him. He was diagnosed with some sort of sexual disorder but I think, he was just a normal teenage boy who hadn't matured yet. At the time of meeting him, he was on the verge of becoming 18 and his consultant was deciding whether to send him to adult PICU or adult rehabilitation. He was in the PICU I was at because he was in general hospital prior for a urinary tract illness. He eventually was issued a catheter which he used to rip out. Obviously, ripping out a catheter can really damage the nether regions and this boy didn't care and was on 2:1 for continuously attempting to rip this out. I remember he kept asking me why I was in hospital and what I did to get there. One time I told him one of my self-harm incidents and he told everyone and embarrassed me. Later, he said that I was attention-seeking when I was listening to my voices. He was unkind but that didn't stop me from wondering what had happened to him.

In the same hospital, was a girl who was 5:1 in the community so 5 staff members would need to accompany her whenever she went out. She got discharged to a hostel because she had nowhere to go. It was sad to think that the doctors overlooked her risk and still let her go even though she was on 5:1!

In the same place was a boy who wasn't ready to be discharged. He used to tell everyone he was fine but I could see in his eyes he wasn't. I know it's weird, but I could tell that he had been through a lot and was still going to do something risky. The night before his discharge, he had a big incident and I knew he wasn't going to be ok. He went anyway and last I heard, he ended up in another unit. I really hope he is still alive today.

In the Low Secure, was a girl who was in general hospital for about 4 months and was being NG tube fed during this time, was IM'd every day and was in restraint every day to the point of needing 4 staff with her. She had to go and have Electro-Convulsive Therapy. She was so kind, timid and genuine. In restraint, she would shout out really loud. She was so institutionalised that she would be scared of going outside, even in the secure garden. She would have breakdowns about this which would lead to restraints.

Once she was in restraint, her state would deteriorate, understandably so; if there were people holding you down, telling you that you couldn't do what you want, it is a given that you are going to become irate and want to get out of being held. It perpetuates further aggression which means you have to be in restraint for longer and it is a cycle which stops when the you get tired- meaning when you are given a tranquiliser injection.

There was another girl, Sky who killed herself after a few months of my discharge. I never expected it. She had BPD, OCD, and an eating disorder.

We used to study together and go horse riding. I hope she is at peace now. I wonder if things would have been different if I had been in touch with her more.

I remember she declared that she was struggling and a staff member (from the Low Secure we were at) said to her that she "looked fine". Well guess what, Mr. Staff Member, she is dead now. She obviously was not fine! I think a lot of professionals may have overlooked her which resulted in her death. It makes me angry that her support team and the medics didn't save her. They have her death on her hands. I am irate, their mistakes cost her life.

I wish people would listen to the miscellaneous mentally ill. Maybe if people did, there wouldn't be so many lives lost.

Chapter 13:

The Challenge of Worth

Staff used to say how he was fine and "didn't need to be in hospital". When people say this, it is incredibly invalidating, as if one has to prove their worth that they need to be in hospital. From what I have observed, it can be a challenge: what is the worst thing you can do to prove you need to be in hospital? It ends up becoming a battle of bravado.

When people say you don't need to be in hospital has many repercussions. It isn't that people want to be in hospital necessarily (although some people do), it is about people saying that you don't belong, it is rejection and being shunned. You can't help being in hospital, especially if you are sectioned, you can't physically remove yourself off section. When people say that you don't need to be in hospital, it is insulting.

Quite often, patients used to approach me and ask me why I was in hospital, saying that they didn't know why I was in hospital because I seemed "normal" or was "too nice to have anything wrong with me". Usually at this, I would plan to do something major to make people understand that I need to be in hospital in a desperate attempt to prove my worth.

It was the same for when professionals would comment on severity of self-harm that wounds are "superficial". This adjective, "superficial" connotes in a young person's mind that their self-harm isn't good enough, isn't grand enough, that they need to do more to get people to validate them and thus, to fell important and worthy.

Everyone needs validation.

When going into hospital, *don't* tell people that they don't need to be in hospital because there are only negative consequences. Everybody is in that place for a reason, respect that.

One example of how these words have a detriment to someone's wellbeing is a boy called Lewis. When I was on his ward, he was quite settled and calm and staff always used to say that he didn't need to be there. Lewis ended up being transferred to a secure forensic unit after staff discovered that he used to cut off heads of rats. This is an extreme example of the lengths people go to in order to feel acceptance and defy others' expectations. It is just unfortunate because he was a clever boy with a lot of potential and people in secure units usually stay there long term so he might have stayed there for a while. It was a pity.

Phase 3:

Miscellaneous

Ramblings of

an Ex-Suicidal

Chapter 14:

The plethora of Psychiatrists

One of my favourite consultant psychiatrists was Dr P. Whenever she was there, we would sing the Dr P song (#Dr P, Dr P, calling Dr P, Dr P, Dr P, get up now!)

She was lovely, just a down-to-earth human being. We were very close and she understood me remarkably well. I used to talk to her about how she used to watch all the TV soaps in medical school- Hollyoaks, Coronation Street, Eastenders, everything. She always used to say how she felt aged 21 in spirit but not in body. Her quirky nature did not stop there, we once conversed about going to the gym and she would day how she had a gym membership which she would use to attend. When I asked her how often she would go, she would say once every few years... She was HILARIOUS-it was funnier because when I asked other staff members, I came to the conclusion that it was true, she truthfully would go to the gym once every 3 years, every year at a push! We shared a common interest in cake.

Other psychiatrists, consisted of the White Witch, of whom I wrote a poem about her:

The White Witch,

My expostulation for *it*

Is explained

It is a lidebound

Logy, lazy liar

Convinced it is a bastion icon

But its lack of erudition stymies my success.

There was also the Smurf doctor. He was a registrar in one hospital and always used to wear this blue shirt and blue jumper and was basically a midget, he was so small and cute. I was very nasty to him but he was good to me, I just didn't see it at the time. He moved on to another hospital, which I ended up going to when I went to PICU, He became a consultant and would wear a full trouser and blouse suit and was very smart but it looked like his clothes were too big for him because of how short and small he was. He was so kind and really tried to listen to what I wanted in my care and I hope he appreciates my gratitude if he is reading this. His name was Dr Billemane but I used to call him the Bacillus which is a rod-shaped bacterium because "he infects people with his lies" as I used to say!

Another one was the Chow. I loathed his existence and state of being with a true passion. He was very inauthentic in his approach towards me and would outright tell me that he was using the ASD positive behaviour approach with me. He was also very judgmental, looking down on me for my dips in religion and spirituality, not to mention being condescending of my relationship with my family. He would refuse to diagnose me with EUPD despite my history of self-harm over a number of years. At one of my gateway assessments to get into inpatient, he asked me if I loved my parents, saying that it was a standard question (it's not!). In his head, he painted me as a weak little girl with ASD with a bit of fake depression. He didn't understand the extent of my illness. His mistake in discharging me nearly cost me my life because I manipulated him into thinking I was fine but within 48 hours of discharge, I had a really big suicide attempt and was sectioned after I had finished treatment for my overdose. He was a horrible man and disregarded many of his patients. I pity the patients who have the misfortune of knowing him. If I had the chance, I would drop him, quicker than he can drop his pants!

There was Dr Potter, I called him "Piss-Pot". In a letter, I called him a "Radix Lecti", which is Latin for couch potato. I said that I hope for ogres to devour his rotting carcass and the goblins bite him in his sleep (or something like that).

Letter to one of my Psychiatrists

One psychiatrist, Madda pressured me into making me speak to my parents. I didn't do it but I deemed it entirely outrageous how she dealt with me. She also stopped my meds to "experiment" (her words) which led to serious deterioration of my mental health to the point where I became psychotic and tried to end my life in a very grave way.

Next up, Dr Madda who said that I might not have EUPD because I had good morals..? (Not all people with EUPD have bad morals!)

I wrote a letter to her, here it goes:

Dearest "Dr",

It feels like the roles are reversed; I have to give you a harangue regarding thinking before speaking. I express no compunction in not being willing to meet your quixotic expectations.

You handled a precarious situation recklessly. My psychological assessment of you is that you show traits of narcissism. You have a cantankerous attitude of inveterate insolence and are pernickety about trivial minutiae. You had the audacity and arrogance to cajole me to do something of which the context is arcane and esoteric. You are ignorant of my true equanimity. You are more a cold, remorseless scientist than a compassionate healthcare professional because you "experiment" with people, as you so magniloquently phrased it yourself.

I won't lionize you, as is the custom, because of your status of being the proverbial "Bossman".

Yours unfortunately,

ZeZe Boi.

Chapter 15:

The Ism Called Autism

I always knew I was different

Never felt like I belonged

Just wanted to be significant

Carried on from childhood and beyond

Years of sensory overloads

Massive meltdowns

Couldn't understand my emotions

Labelled the "difficult child"

Not until the doctor came around

When I was shouting and sobbing on the ground

She asked lots of questions after sitting me down,

"Why are you asking me that, you noisy cow?"

Eventually she said, "Autism"

"What is this -ism?"

"Isn't that what old people get?"

"Is it contagious?"

No, no, no she said

You see the world in a different way

You find it hard to make a friend

For you it is black-and-white, there is no grey

You are different but it should be celebrated!

We all deserve to be accepted as we are

You're like a cake in a cookie jar

Don't be frustrated, be belated

You're a unicorn in a field of horses

The neuordiverse should unite as special force

Chapter 16:

Autism

When I was first diagnosed with Asperger's Syndrome (Autism) I thought it was something old people got, a type of dementia. I had no idea what it meant which was quite scary. What was horrible was that at the time, I was in the pre-suicidal phase and I wasn't looking for an autism diagnosis, I was looking for a mental health diagnosis which explained how I felt the way I did.

Upon reflection, I do agree I have it but I have grown out of it over the years- I am (it is politically incorrect but) only a little bit autistic. It doesn't affect me too much now. I don't get sensory overloads very much anymore, I am ok with crowds, eye contact. I find it difficult to talk a lot and be sociable but I am working on it. I have coping skills now and ways I handle things.

Thinking back to when I was younger, there probably were moments where I can identify as being admittedly a bit autistic.

A prime example is when I was in primary school. One night, my dad was talking to me about the Muslim prophet (peace be upon him) and how he didn't like proud people and that it was a bad quality as it led to arrogance. The next day, my teacher picked me to be school council and I went to the head-teacher's office to collect my badge. She gave us a speech about how we were ambassadors of the school and we should wear the badge with pride. Immediately, at this, I shook my head and said how I couldn't be proud, wasn't allowed to. The teachers questioned if I wanted to do it and said that they could ask someone else to be school council if I wished. I did want to be school council, it was just that my dad told me to never be proud and I took that literally. Me taking this literally and remembering the exact words my dad said was an early sign of my autism rearing its head. My neurodivergence meant that I had difficulty understanding language and interpreted it very differently. The teacher obviously meant that I should be proud of doing school council and my dad was simply telling me to be a good person and to never be arrogant. I misunderstood this. I was too young at the time to verbalise this and understand what that meant. It is only now that I get it.

Another example is of when I was younger, I used to hate being touched. It was a sensory thing which I used to absolutely hate the feeling of up until I was about 17. I can deal with it now. At school, the teacher tapped me on the shoulder telling me well done. I hated this and due to my sensory issues, it felt more than just a tap because of my hypersensitivity. This really upset me and made me feel uncomfortable. The teacher wasn't doing anything wrong, it was just that I couldn't deal with people touching, it was not done with ill intent. When I went home, I told my parents the teacher touched me and that I hated it. It got brought to the head-teacher's attention as a safeguarding issue and it was misunderstood by the people around me and I wasn't able to explain what I meant due to being so young. In actuality, it was just a sensory problem rather than me making a false allegation.

Looking back at my life, I can see how I had black and white thinking, I was unable to comprehend facial expressions and struggled with change.

When I was about 9, my family got a new car and I cried the whole journey home because I wanted to get a different car and I couldn't cope with the change. I was miserable.

Another change I struggled to cope with was when I was going into reception and primary school. I would cry for my mum to pick me up from school until I was in year 3. I would pretend to have tummy aches and would be adamant that I needed to go home. The transition to school was really difficult for me and I would cry for hours at school. No teacher could console me, I was defiantly moody.

Autism presents differently in boys. Girls have an internalising psychopathology. It goes back to gender roles in society. If a boy is upset, stereotypically, they will fight it out. If a girl is upset, she probably won't outright say it but internalise it. Girls, from a young age, are able to mask their difficulties in order to blend in with society. This doesn't come as naturally to men, not at all in a sexist way. Here is some research to back this up:

(Michelle Dean, Robin Harwood, Connie Kasari)

"The results indicate that the female social landscape supports the camouflage hypothesis; girls with autism spectrum disorder used compensatory behaviors, such as staying in close proximately to peers and weaving in and out of activities, which appeared to mask their social challenges. Comparatively, the male landscape made it easier to detect the social challenges of boys with autism spectrum disorder. Typically developing boys tended to play organized games; boys with autism spectrum disorder tended to play alone. The results highlight a male bias in our perception of autism spectrum disorder. If practitioners look for social isolation on the playground when identifying

children with social challenges, then our findings suggest that girls with autism spectrum disorder will continue to be left unidentified."

I think this is why it took so long for me to get diagnosed with autism. I masked my difficulties and was just thought to be really sensitive and I had to have people explain things to me in a way that I would understand.

Now, nobody can tell that I have autism unless you spent a significant amount of time with me. It is an invisible disorder. Whenever I speak with people and tell them that I have autism, they would never guess it and I am told that I am really not autistic. I can even comprehend metaphors, which some autistic people can't get to terms with.

Chapter 17:

Attachment Schema

During my course of schema CBT therapy, I discovered, alongside my therapist, that I probably had an attachment issue when I was younger. This would relate to why I would cry for my mum at school until I was in year 3.

I also developed a schema that I wasn't lovable due to when my father told me I had 2 half-brothers from a previous marriage. This was my first episode of experiencing rejection. I felt as if my dad loved me less because if he now had 6 children to share his love between, instead of just 4, it meant he had less love for me. It was also due to my autism and attachment issues that I thought my dad loved me less now that I had 2 half-brothers. I think this was why I really struggled to talk to my dad sometimes. When I would be on the ward, I remember my mum asked me why I hadn't seen my dad in a while. It was because whenever I experienced rejection, I would want to avoid my dad because he was the first person I felt rejected me and I didn't want to be around him to remember that.

My attachment problems were not limited to this. When I was 12, my first psychologist, Katharine left for another job and her departure fuelled my depression and poor self-esteem. I thought I had done something wrong to make her want to leave. This made my mental health deteriorate further and it was around that time that I first started being admitted into general hospital for feeling suicidal. Her leaving made me want to die.

The more I delved into the mental health system, in inpatient and outpatient, my attachment problems spiralled. I remember, in my residential children's home, when staff left, I would be really upset. This would happen a lot because it is natural in care for there to be a high staff turnover. When a support worker of whom I was close with, left, I tried to kill myself and ended up having a fifth hospital admission that lasted 1 and a half years. Nobody understood how I got to the point I did and why my mental state had deteriorated. Nobody could understand and my house manager was grappling for reasons as to why my risk behaviour had increased so much. She even said I got "emotionally dysregulated due to staff not giving me halal chicken". But no, it was because a staff member left and I couldn't cope with it, the feeling of worthlessness got so intense and I thought that I deserved to die because of her leaving.

Secure attachments (for me) meant that it would take a long time for me to trust someone and when I did, I would think of them as my "forever" people, people who would always be there for me and love me regardless. I had an ambivalent attachment which meant that I was always looking for validation and approval. My self-worth was based off if those people cared about me. Constantly, I would find accuse them (Staff) of not caring because I needed them to tell me that they loved and care for me.

I even wrote a letter in my own blood to a staff member when a staff member, who I was close to, announced they were leaving. I ended up not giving it to them because I was soon placed under a section 3 after this. I did this because I wanted them to feel a fraction of the pain I felt, the void that they left in my heart and how I didn't want to be alive without them in my life.

Throughout my fifth admission, I tried to talk about my attachment problems. I used to tell staff that I wanted to stop talking to them because I didn't want to get close to them because I knew that, if I kept talking to them, I would end up becoming even more suicidal and I knew the relationships with staff in hospitals are not permanent and that it would come to an end at some point so I didn't want the unnecessary heartbreak.

Chapter 18:

Nanny McPhee paradox

I also think that one of my schemas was that I needed to be risky to be cared for which probably added to my attachment problems. In hospital, I would be risky and staff would tell me that they cared about me and wanted me to get better, they would tell me I had a bright future and that they were going to be there for me. Eventually I got in the habit of self-harming in order to incite a care response. This was an autism thing, said the professionals but I think this goes deeper than autism. When I was in some of the darkest places, I felt cared for. For example, when I was put on 3:1 and 2:1 (where 3 or 2 people would have to be within arms-reach of me to stop me from hurting myself, running away or hitting people) I was suicidal, but felt like people understood me and would care for me. That feeling of being understood was really comforting and validating because I never felt like I was understood. People spent time with me and put measures in place to ensure I was supported. When I was doing well and about to be discharged, people were not like this to me, quite the opposite, they would leave me alone to my own devices and I didn't feel loved or appreciated.

Unfortunately, that is just how the system works, when patients are risky, staff have to support them and comfort them because they need it but when they are ok and in recovery, staff naturally don't spend as much time with them because they don't need it, seemingly.

When staff were with me, keeping me safe from hurting myself, I wouldn't like them, I wouldn't like being on 2:1 or 3:1 but in hindsight, now that I am doing well, I wish I had that care response.

It is like Nanny McPhee, when I needed staff to keep me safe (but didn't want them to keep me safe), I would hate them but when I wanted them to keep me safe (but didn't *need* them to keep me safe), I would miss them because they would leave.

Chapter 18: Hallucinations and Delusions

Yes, I heard voices. No, I wasn't possessed. No, I didn't murder anyone. I was just very unwell.

My first episodes was following a major depressive episode. Later on, it was concluded that due to my BPD, when I got stressed, I would get psychotic. This would mean hearing voices, seeing apparitions, paranoia and having delusions. It was a very dark time.

I would see very graphic and vivid people, sometimes they would be floating, and sometimes they would be on the floor and dead. My voices were so clear in my head but it felt like they came from above so whenever I would listen to them, I would look up because that was where I thought they were coming from.

My delusions included thinking people were Jesus, that I was in purgatory instead of hospital, that walls had portals (as well as plug sockets) and that I had killed a baby.

When I was paranoid, I would get people to taste-test my food to ensure there was no poison or trackers in what I was eating. This went on for about 6-9 months. I would only eat packet food because I would know this wasn't contaminated. My voices used to tell me that if I didn't hurt myself, they would kill people that I cared about. My psychosis also manifested itself in terms of me not sleeping. I would go a week without sleeping because I was convinced somebody would attack me in my sleep. The longer I stopped sleeping, the worse my psychosis got. This meant that on the wards, I would sleep in the lounge because I knew there were cameras there and people would get caught if they did anything to me. It was like this for 3 months. I did also have a stage where I was running at walls thinking that they were a portal to Narnia, leading to a big hematoma on my head and needing restraint. I thought if I put my fingers in plug sockets, this would also send me to Narnia.

There is nothing scarier than not being able to trust your mind, but then not being able to trust others too. It is frightening when people are telling you that the things you see are not real. Whenever I would talk about my beliefs and delusions, the psychiatrists would just say, "I believe you believe that," when they really thought I was just really unwell. It makes you wonder: if that isn't real, what constitutes reality? I constantly felt like the world around me was a simulation, not real. The world simply seemed superficial. In every corner my mind delved into, there was an aura of uncertainty. I felt like my mind was walking a tight rope between insanity and my perception of reality.

Despite this, I managed to find some sort of comfort in my voices- they were there for me when nobody else could be. They kept me company. I was friends with my own voices. Despite the pain I endured at their hand, I needed them for validation. I guess this was part of me collapsing on myself, retreating into my Mind Palace. I kept the walls to my Mind Palace so high that the only type of communication I would allow would be with my voices.

Chapter 19: Palace Analogy

The palace analogy refers to a concept I would refer to when talking about my difficulty trusting.

Figuratively, I have a palace, a Mind Palace. For the most part, I do not allow people in this palace. It has sky high walls, strengthened over the course of years by bricks and barricades fastened to the sharp portcullis. I test people to determine if they are trustworthy over the course of months. They give me the façade that they are to be trusted, ergo, I let them in, at which point they bring in their mob of strangers with blades and pitchforks. They torch my palace, wreck it, steal and smash my belongings and ornaments. They leave me to watch my palace, everything I work so hard to build, to go up in flames. I am left with an empty, abandoned wreck of a building and I put all my energies into security and building walls even higher than before.

The worst of it is that I would feel so guilty for letting these people in in the first place!

This is a metaphor for when people I meet leave me and I feel so suicidal that this is how I feel. I wrote staff letters in my blood so that they could understand a fraction of the kind of pain I feel.

Chapter 21:

The Lessons I Learnt

During my journey to recovery, there were a few lessons I had to learn. Each skill took a long time to master and for me to get used to. I write these in the hope that other people can use these as coping strategies like me

- People are never going to be the people I want them to be. I can expect people to be the depiction of all that is good in the world, but in reality, nobody is perfect, everybody has a fatal flaw, it's tragic but true. This rings true for everyone, from friends to professionals to family. My walls may be high but I don't need to have expectations as high. This means I don't have to over-idealise a relationship then be bitterly disappointed with the real deal. Aim low, get high.
- All relationships have a purpose. There is a variety of people in the world, there are those who you play an imperative role and some who might not be so prevalent. Not everybody in my life are going to be there forever. Even the strangers who hold the door for me on my way to school have a role to play in my life. No matter how short term a relationship is, that person may bring joy into my life, even if it is just for a day. I don't have to close my Mind Palace to people because I know they are going to leave me. I don't have to have a sharp portcullis with unbreakable ivy wrapped around it and a series of cannons ready for if people try to enter. Even the briefest encounters with people could bring something extra to my life. I don't have to shut myself off even though that has been my protective factor for years.
- Gratitude is important. Many a time, I have had staff or family say to me that I need to stop being selfish and throwing my life away because people in hospitals and disadvantaged countries fight for their life, meanwhile, here I am trying to end it all. I have heard people say to people with eating disorders that they are not eating but people in disadvantaged countries (everybody always says Africa, but Africa is a vast continent, not a country and some parts of Africa are actually quite prosperous!) would fight for that food. Although the sentiment is there, the understanding is not. Yes, gratitude is important but it shouldn't be adapted to this situation. Being grateful should make someone feel better about their position, not guilty for feeling or behaving the way they do. I have a gratitude journal that I write in every so often. I keep it

to feel better about my position. Gratitude helps me not to wallow into self-despair.

- It is ok to be in the middle.
  I know there are more people I have met that I haven't mentioned and who might not have been one of the few I chose to trust but were still civil to me but I find it difficult to recognise this because due to my diagnoses. I am a very extreme person and think of people as either good or bad, with no happy medium. This is why I haven't mentioned everybody I have met during my admissions. Although I am grateful for everything they have done for me, but I have only mentioned the people who were particularly special to me. It is one of my flaws and I am working on it. It took me a while to realise that I don't have over-idealise someone or bluntly catastrophize my relationship with them. Those are 2 dialectics and it is possible to find a middle path. This is ostensibly easier said than done.

- I don't have to like someone for them to support me. Liking people helps but isn't always needed. With real life people, friends and such, it is a different story but with professionals, they are there to care for me- that's their job! I don't have to like them in order to access that care, otherwise they are unprofessional. It is their job to care for all their patients, not just the ones they take favour to.
- Reality test it.
  Reality testing has proved a very important skill for me to use when I have crises. It is used to compare my internal thoughts with external reality. I start with identifying an initial thought and then twisting it to adapt to reality. For example, my initial thought could be: People don't care about me. (This is a thought which always crops up when my mental health starts to deteriorate.) My reality test would be: People wouldn't have asked if I was ok repeatedly if they didn't care. They wouldn't have tried to have a chat with me or engage with me. This really helps me to rationalise my thoughts.
- Writing letters to my future self helps. Here is one:

Dear Future Self,

If you are reading this, it is because you are suicidal again and need your past self to remind how far you have come.

I want you to be happy. You don't deserve this pain. You are worthy of love, you are worthy of life. You have fought too hard to give up now.

Mental illness is not who you are. Humans are complex forms with many, many layers and the state of mental health is in no way connected to identity.

Everybody has mental health issues, the same way that everybody has physical health issues from time to time. Mental health is health.

It is not uncommon to have bad days, days where you can't be bothered to get out of bed or when you cry for a whole day following a distressing event. This is something everybody encounters at some stage. Anybody and everybody can find themselves in a less-than-ideal situation. Hardship is inevitable, albeit unpleasant, but a necessary part of the human experience.

Yes, you have been through a lot and right now, you might feel broken. But you don't have to say broken. Suicide is fixing a temporary problem with a permanent solution. If you die, nothing will get better, if you stay, there is a chance it will.

If you are looking for a sign not to kill yourself, this is it.

Love yourself.

Your Past Self.

- Validation checks.
  Validation is something that I have struggled to receive and input myself. This manifested itself in the form of insecure attachments (in layman terms, I struggled with relationships in my life because of this)
  There is 2 types of validation that I have skills for; validation of others and self-validation.
  Validation of others means to accept someone else's point of view- you don't necessarily have to agree, just acknowledge their opinion to fulfil their sense of approval. For example, I might not agree with my family's view on my fashion sense, I don't agree with them but I accept that this is their view.
  This is what I would say to my family: I know this may be difficult to hear. I know that you care for me, as my family and want me to look my best. You are always looking out for me and I appreciate that. I would like to wear clothes that I like, I am more independent and would like to make these decisions myself and I still value your opinion.

Here is the checklist:

1. Acknowledge the potential difficulty in them hearing your response: e.g. this might be difficult for you to hear
2. Acknowledge the value or intensity of the other person's advice or point of view: e.g. I want you to know I really value your advice.
3. Guess the emotion the other person is experiencing and their intention for communicating with you: e.g. I can see that you are worried about me.
4. State your position: e.g. I disagree/hold a different view
5. I agree partially: e.g. although I haven't changed my mind, it has helped me think of ways that I can better manage a situation.

Now for self-validation.

I am, like most people in life, quite harsh on myself and often forget to be kind to myself and practise self-care and self-love. This is not a "hippy-dippy" topic, it is an important part of functioning, especially if an individual is unable to receive validation from other people. It is like food; if other people can't make it for you, you have to do it yourself, cook for yourself. If you don't cook for yourself, you can become malnourished and unwell. At the end of the day, it is something you have to do in order to be the best version of yourself that you can be. Self-love is no different. Some people have too much and indulge in food and this dual meaning of obesity from nutrition and obesity of self-love can turn into arrogance and has negative consequences. If there is too little, you can become starved of self-esteem. Validation of one's self is essential in feeling confident.

Here is how to self-validate:

1. Connect with the emotion/thoughts/judgements that you are experiencing. E.g. I am noticing I am feeling sad
2. Validate and acknowledge the presence of these motions. Thoughts and judgments. E.g. it is ok to feel angry.
3. What might you say to someone else experiencing this emotion
4. Reflect on past experiences to encourage and empower yourself in the moment. E.g. I remember a time when I wasn't able to do this and I can see the progress I have made.
5. What can you learn from this emotion? What action can you take now or in the future when you are calm? E.g. what is it about this that is making me feel angry?

6. How can I turn this into a positive experience? E.g. thinking having gone through this experience I am now stronger.

I find it easier to write all the above down so that I can read it to myself. I write it as if I am writing it to someone else because this helps me to be less self-critical. If I were to write this up for someone else, I would put more compassion in it then if it were to be myself.

- Self-care isn't selfish. There are a variety of ways that people self-regulate by doing things they enjoy in order to relax. For me, watching Netflix is how I switch off. It isn't lazy or wasting time as long as it doesn't consume all my time and I am still being productive. All people need to do things that help them to relax and switch off. That can be by doing something conventionally related to self-care such as meditation or something like taking a walk. Anything you enjoy that enables you to "switch off" will be beneficial. Ideally, this should be done every day or every week. Taking time for yourself to preserve your mental state is never a sign of laziness or selfishness.
- Since, I have learnt that I am allowed to be happy. It is not selfish to be happy. I have proved to myself I am able to be happy in the long term and sustain it.

Chapter 22:

Borderline Personality Disorder

Borderline Personality Disorder or Emotionally Unstable Personality Disorder is one of the most stigmatised illnesses, not just for people with this illness but also for professionals working with patients with this. BPD is Diagnosis of exclusion. It is one of the least understood illnesses ad each medic I have met and has had a different view on it.

"Borderline personality disorder (BPD) is characterised by a pattern of instability of interpersonal relationships, self-image and affects, and by marked impulsivity. Its diagnosis does not imply any specific cause. BPD is defined descriptively, in terms of its associated impairments. There are two main sets of diagnostic criteria in current use, the International Classification of Mental and Behavioural Disorders 10th Revision (ICD-10) and the Diagnostic and Statistical Manual of Mental Disorders fourth edition (DSM-IV). ICD-10 uses the term emotionally unstable personality disorder, dividing this into two variants (impulsive type and borderline type) both of which share the general theme of impulsiveness and lack of self-control. The impulsive variant is characterised by a tendency to conflict and outbursts of anger or violence, difficulty in maintaining any course of action that offers no immediate reward, and instability of mood; the borderline variant is characterised by disturbances of self-image, a tendency to unstable relationships, efforts to avoid abandonment, and threats or acts of self-harm (including suicide). In DSM-IV, BPD is defined more broadly to include all of the features of the borderline variant of emotionally unstable personality disorder and most of the criteria for the impulsive variant. DSM-IV also defines all personality disorders as axis II BPD final scope 02 03 07. Page 2 of 11 disorders. BPD is defined as a cluster B disorder ('dramatic, emotional or erratic' type) along with antisocial, histrionic and narcissistic personality disorders. There is substantial comorbidity of borderline personality disorder (BPD) with common mental disorders such as depressive illness, the range of anxiety disorders or substance misuse disorders. d) There is some divergence between ICD-10 and DSM-IV as to whether borderline/emotionally unstable personality disorder can be diagnosed in those younger than 18 years, and this may lead to uncertainties about the usage of the diagnosis in young people. In ICD-10 the disorder comes within the overall grouping of disorders of adult personality and behaviour, but DSM-IV specifies that BPD can be diagnosed in those younger than 18 if the features of the disorder have been present for at least 1 year." (NICE guidelines)

The Stigma of BPD

One might think that there is no longer stigma against people with mental health problems, surely we have moved past that…this is true- but not for people with BPD.

People with PD are thought of as "manipulative". No, we are just bad at interpersonal effectiveness. Everybody manipulates to get what they want out of life. Asking someone at college for help with homework is manipulative because I am using someone to get what I want. Neurotypicals don't call this manipulative because of the way this is done (e.g. if you say please and thank you to the person and butter them up a bit by complementing them: "You are super clever and I want to be like you so please could you help me with my homework.")This is manipulation but because it is done well, it is just thought of as good communication rather than manipulation.

So do people with PD, except, we will say things like, "If you don't do this for me, I will kill myself," This is not accepted in society and is an example of ineffective communication, thus is thought of negatively and labelled "manipulation".

Then there is the commonly used adjective that is used to describe people with this illness; "attention-seeking". First of all, everybody in life needs attention to some extent. BPD can be thought of as attention-seeking because we crave validation due to being not given this in the past. We have a desperate need to be understood.

People need to understand that this behaviour is not borne out of malice or ill intent, but out of being unwell. This is how the illness manifests itself.

A nurse from one of my PICUs told me that he had known a psychiatrist who told him that BPD is not an illness, it is part of someone's everyday functioning and who they are. Some of the behaviours that BPD people present with are deemed unacceptable in society (such as self-harm) which is why people give them this label. They thought BPD was just a reaction to traumatic life experiences. It was an interesting theory.

A psychiatrist lent me a book which said that BPD is the line between neurotic (psychiatric conditions such as anxiety and depression) and psychotic illnesses which is why it is called "borderline". This is no longer true. This is the old view of BPD. It is now thought of as being emotionally unstable (Hence it being called "Emotionally Unstable Personality Disorder")

In this way, most professionals have different perspectives on the illness. There is a lot of controversy about it. Personally, I think that the diagnosis shouldn't be scrapped because if I didn't have that diagnosis, I wouldn't have had any treatment or gone to the Low Secure which later saved my life.

My BPD affects me in the following ways:

- Attachment problems and scared of rejection or termination of relationships. Frantic efforts to avoid abandonment by others. Endings are really difficult. I once wrote a letter to staff members in my blood so that they could feel the same pain I did- I thought this was the best way to deal with this at the time. In hospital, I would be nasty to staff but only because I wanted to push them away because I didn't want to get close to people because I knew that the relationship would end and that I would end up feeling suicidal once they left my life. It was very complex. It was the "I Hate You, Don't Leave Me" effect. This would mean: "I will leave you before you leave me", "I will hate you before you hate me".
- Intense relationships with others-shifting from idealising to detesting. I have to work 5 times harder when it comes to relationships. Either want to be really close or have nothing to do with people.
- Chronic Suicidality and self-harm
- Unstable sense of self- not knowing who I want to be and fluctuating core values e.g. not wanting to be Muslim
- Low self-esteem. -pure hatred of myself and self-loathing. I wholeheartedly believed I was a horrible disgusting human being and deserved the worst treatment. Internally I just wanted to be loved and validated.
- Intense moods. I feel emotions all-encompassing and very strongly.
- Intense and inappropriate outbursts of anger. When I am angry, I write horrible hate mail to people which involve death threats and really nasty insults. I told my psychologist that I hope goblins consume her rotting

carcass. It is really harsh but at the time, I whole-heartedly mean it because of how furious I am. It is a dysfunctional way of coping because when I send these letters, it can result in breaking off relationships.

- Episodes of paranoid thoughts, psychotic symptoms and dissociation in times of stress. Psychotic episodes and paranoid delusions. Had to get other people to taste my food to ensure I didn't get poisoned. Would think there were snipers out to get me, that my doctor would assault me.

BPD or a response to Trauma?

BPD is usually a response to trauma. It goes back to the schema therapy model where there is an assumption that events that happen in your early life can affect our core beliefs or actions in the present day. It doesn't necessarily have to be a severely traumatic experience, could be anything slightly negative. For example, there was someone I know who said that once they got stuck in a public toilet for 3 hours after the lock broke and only got out after a cleaner opened the door. From then on, that person no longer locked the toilet behind her. People would always barge in, thinking it was empty but she would be sat there on the toilet, refusing to lock the door. She would rather be embarrassed and have people walk in then to relive the experience of having the door locked. It says a lot. This kind of thing happens to everyone. Now apply it to someone who has encountered a traumatic experience- it would affect your future decisions and behaviour, every aspect of life! It shows that early life experiences always shape the people we become.

With personality disorder, these life experiences are usually traumatic or adverse to the point that we become unable to regulate our emotions successfully and so we turn to socially unacceptable behaviours to cope and self-soothe, such as self-harm. It isn't just emotion dysregulation that get affected, but every aspect of life, such as interpersonal effectiveness and distress tolerance.

I Hate You Don't Leave Me Effect

This is the title to a song which I would say is the BPD anthem.

"I'm addicted to the madness

I'm a daughter of the sadness

I've been here too many times before

Been abandoned and I'm scared now

I can't handle another fall out

I'm fragile, just washed upon the shore

They forget me, don't see me

When they love me, they leave me"

This perfectly encapsulates the struggles of a borderline. I thought that I was attached to being in hospital as it was a safe place. I thought depression and suicidality was engraved in my heart and it was just part of me that wasn't going to change. I used to be very emotionally fragile and people would have to walk on eggshells around me-my parents did this for years. I don't mean fragile like a little flower, I mean fragile like a bomb waiting to implode. When I would get to know staff at hospital, they would love me and come to understand me but eventually, they would "leave me" because I would be discharged or transferred to another hospital. It was damaging.

It was the "I Hate You, Don't Leave Me" effect. This would mean: "I will leave you before you leave me", "I will hate you before you hate me", and "I will hurt you before you hurt me".

It was a hard cycle to get out of, taking almost a year of intensive therapy!

Chapter 23:

Being comfortable with Hospital life

I think there are some people in hospital of whom will remain there for a large period of time. I knew a girl who used to swallow very large foreign objects (including utensils!) in my Low Secure. She had so much potential- she was intelligent (working towards getting her GCSEs) and kind (she used to always be there for people when they were feeling down or having a wobble). She was brilliant and a real pleasure to be around... but every couple of months, she would have these major incidents from which she would need surgery and be placed on 2:1 in a sterilised room. It was so sad because when she was doing so well, she wanted nothing more than to continue building a life worth living for herself. Her EUPD (which might have been Complex PTSD also) meant that she would impulsively do things and sometimes regret this later. She was on 1:1, no bathroom privacy for about 2 years. She had a very dark past, her birth parents abused her as a child and did some horrible things to her and she was adopted by another family who were not entirely supportive of her struggles. This is a prime example of someone who might stay in hospital for a long, long time. Once she has come to terms with her past and once she has accessed the right therapeutic interventions, she will flourish. I really hope she will be able to move on eventually.

Sometimes, people who have spent a long time in hospital are scared of getting better. This is a common occurrence for people with complex illnesses. There were a girl I met who was scared of even stepping a foot outside because she hadn't gone out in the real world for years due to being institutionalised. She was just 15.

"Why would people be scared to get better?" you ask. There are many reasons. It could be because individuals are not used to being happy because they have been depressed for such a long time. It could be because when someone is quite far gone in their recovery, mental health services withdraw their support, and for someone with attachment issues or fear of abandonment, this is something very difficult to cope with. It could be because people see no hope and the idea of recovery seems so daunting and unfamiliar that even thinking about recovery overloads them. Things are a lot more complex than you'd think. It could be that in hospital, staff care for you, they feed you, give you shelter, do all the cleaning for you, to the point that going out in the real world doesn't seem enough. A lot of daily chores and opportunities to be independent are stripped away. Ostensibly, when people reach the stage of discharge, it is extremely difficult, even debilitating, to get used to "real life".

If everything you need is in hospital, what is the point of leaving it? Life is too difficult anyway.

That is how some people think and feel. Mental illness is incredibly complex, it goes deeper than just feeling a bit sad. There is always more to a story.

Chapter 24:

Groove Theory

The way I see these kinds of complex cases is that, when someone has been in hospital for a long time and has built a list of maladaptive coping strategies (e.g. self-harm), it is as if their mind has built a groove into the neural pathway. If something happened, your mind would fall in to the groove of feeling a certain way or reacting in a certain way. For example, if someone were to experience a hardship in life, their groove would mean they would behave in a certain way by (for example), self-harming. This is more common with people with Emotionally Unstable Personality Disorder from what I have observed. We, EUPDs (Emotionally Unstable Personality Disorder), have a pattern of self-harming and self-destructive behaviour over the long term and it becomes normal to us to use self-harm as a coping strategy, so much that it becomes second nature.

It is much harder to carve a new path to develop positive coping strategies because of this groove. If EUPDs were to actively attempt to break this self-harm cycle, it would prove a lot more difficult. Instead of self-harming when a situation arises, and we were to replace it with (For example), going to the gym, it would be a lot less natural and wouldn't have the same effect as it would if self-harm was done instead.

It is similar to how someone might try to eat slightly healthier. Instead of reaching for a packet of crisps, you might chew on carrot sticks. It doesn't taste as good at first, but after a while, you get used to it and your taste buds adjust. It is just like that but with self-harm instead. When trying to get out of that cycle, you have to use another strategy- it might not satisfy that self-harm urge and might not work for the first few weeks or months, whilst you carve a new "groove" into your brain. Eventually that groove will become less artificial. It may take a while but one day it will feel natural to use a new coping strategy.

Chapter 25:

A Restrictive Way of Life

I have now been in and out of hospital for 4 years. I came into psychiatric units at the age of 14 and am now approaching 18. I still feel 14 because of the years I have missed out on, being locked away in institutions. It changed me. Slowly, life began to adapt to me being in hospital. Everything worked around it.

Being away from family meant that I, unknowingly, built a support network of staff members whom all later became my surrogate family. They would be there for me when I needed support the most. Whether it be tears, laughter or sighs of boredom, it would be shared with support workers and nurses. People who knew everything about me- from the way I had a cup of tea to my darkest secrets. These people knew everything about me.

Hospital worked around other stuff in different ways. Eventually, it became the norm to have pat downs after leaving the ward, going out on leave or just routine pat downs. Some people had pat downs before and after going to the toilet.

When coming back from leave, staff would take staples from inside magazines, any items considered to be contraband would be thrown, locked away and forgotten about in some cupboards. They would take ring binder wires from books.

People became accustomed to rules such as wearing non-wired sports bras (as the wire was contraband), wearing ankle socks (as normal socks were a risk), using hair removal cream instead of shaving (because razors were contraband, ostensibly).

TV's were locked away in a transparent box; wardrobes and bathrooms were locked; pens were contraband and utilising them was only done so with close supervision. Some people were supervised 2:1 to use a pen or knit. Others, were too risky to have paper. Even toilet paper was limited for some people.

Windows either opened with a grate of little holes to let the air through or they opened a mere inch.

Only 2 teddies, 2 books and 3 pens were allowed to be out in my room. Only settled people could have curtains. Blue tac was contraband so posters were stuck up with glue dots or masking tape (because normal tape was also contraband). Wrappers from food and clothes tags were contraband.

Food was served to use through a hatch, a hole in wall, which was only just big enough to let a plastic plate go through. We had plastic crockery. Food was served to us at fixed times during the day. We were expected to be on ward, and be dressed at exact times.

Housekeepers did all the cleaning that needed to be done because we were not allowed access to cleaning products for obvious reasons.

There was limited Computer Access. The news, soaps and social media was banned. Words such as "butterfly" and "scrapbook" were flagged up as inappropriate because it had the words "butt" and "crap" in.

It was a norm to refrain from having your head covered by the duvet because when the staff came to check on me, they would have to peel back the covers to see my face-they had to do "face checks". A lot of the time, they needed to see my hands too.

I haven't even made a cup of tea for myself in 2 years.

People would kick off or "display behaviours" at least 4 times a day.

With all this in mind, it is easy to see how regimental hospital life was. The measures to keep us safe was excessive, yet necessary for some. Yes, it was incredibly restrictive and isolated but it was just something patients had to get used to. If anything, it was an incentive for people to want to move on from inpatient settings.

Being in the community now, without all these restrictions is very strange. It is hard to adjust from coming from a very extreme environment. Now, I can make drinks whenever I want, I don't need to ask to go to the toilet and have staff unlock the door. I can write whenever I want without having to be supervised with a pen for only 30 minutes at a time. I am allowed to books with a ring binder to just freely sit in my flat, not locked in a contraband cupboard. People are not checking on me every 5 or every 15 minutes. Real life is completely different.

Chapter 26:

Fybogel

Fybogel is an important aspect to my recovery. I wake up every morning, and when I struggle to find reasons to get up, I just think, "Yes, I can have Fybogel". It is most definitely, the highlight to my day. At present, I have wangled my way into having it be prescribed a whopping 2 times a day-BONUS! I approach each Fybogel does with gusto and deep-rooted appreciation. This delicacy gives me life purpose. The most refreshing flavour is Orange (lemon is for wimps). It brings inner contentment. I would like to profess my gratitude towards whosoever was gifted enough as to invent this.

Thank you. It is truly an experience. May God bless your soul.

When nurses ask me what other medication I have other than Fybogel, I reply with, "Nothing else is as important as fybogel, besides that is my day to day shit."

#Isaphagula

Chapter 27:

Dirty Protests

Once I knew a boy, Zahid. He was on the same High Dependency Unit as me and he was psychotic. The anti-psychotics they put him on made him eat excessively and he had to get a dietician to help him to stop him becoming obese.

One day, I woke up to a strange smell in my room...I wondered out of my room and through the ward towards the Communal Area. Everybody, like me, had gathered to figure out what it was, the stench grew stronger and stronger. Rumour was, Zahid had wiped his own poo all over his bedroom. All we could see were nurses going in and out of his room with dirty wipes, surgical face masks and yellow aprons. Apparently, he had smeared it all over his bedroom walls and the staff had to clean it all up, using a jet wash and steamer for infection control. The stench...it was potent, like baby poo. I know that may sound mean, but from what we could smell, it must have been a runny poo...

That wasn't even the worst of it.

On a later date, I was in the Communal Area, waiting for the teachers to come for "Drop Everything and Read" club when I heard footsteps pattering along laminate flooring. I thought nothing of it. Mindlessly looking up, I glanced it was Zahid naked...what-he was naked?!?! I didn't even look again, I didn't know where to look, I covered my eyes, my mouth dropped and all I could hear was the sound of his chilling laugh. All of a sudden, I heard the pattering feet come closer...Oh crap! (Pun intended) He was running after me. I took off, trying to get away from, we ran around the sofas and through the corridors, I was shouting out for help for a nurse- a naked boy was running after me!!!!

"HELP! I NEED A NURSE!"

All the nurses were dispensing medication? What do I do, he was going to get me and probably do something to me!!

Thankfully, the staff on 1:1 observations observed this and stopped him from getting to me!

Phew!

That was a close one.

One of the patients who witnessed that told me that he had his own poo all over his hands and he was trying to wipe it on me- GROSS! It makes me shudder just thinking about it!

Another time, he hugged me from the back and tried to...do stuff...I felt violated...it was vile behaviour and I shouldn't have to be subjected to that however I understand that he was ill and couldn't control his actions.

These kinds of things are rare-patients are not usually subjected to these kinds of behaviours unless it is on a PICU (Psychiatric Intensive Care Unit) or HDU (High Dependency Unit).

Talking of psychotic behaviour, in one of my PICUs, there was a boy who used to hit staff every day, without fail, at the same time, he had schizoaffective disorder and autism. He used to spit at staff a lot, and sometimes, his spit would reach some of the patients-it was disgusting- I know he couldn't help it and was mentally unwell but at the same time, it is far from pleasant to be on the receiving end of this.

There was another boy who used to lay on the floor, making sexual noises for at least an hour straight, without a break, in the communal area, blocking the way to the office. He was so loud, it was impossible to block it out. When he was well, he had no recollection of this and was actually quite reserved and shy. He had bipolar disorder and got psychotic when he was manic.

A girl called Flute, used to dance on table tops and run into rooms, screaming, "I can see the fairies!"

Another girl used to strip when she was manic.

A boy once slapped an old male nurse's bum. He used to roll up playing cards and put it in his mouth, pretending it was a cigarette and that he was smoking some sort of illicit drug (his psychosis was drug induced). He used to tell all the female support workers that he was in love with them and wanted to marry them. He told me I was possessed and that my pseudo-hallucinations were demons. NOT. HELPFUL. He couldn't help it though.

It is sad to see how dire people get when they experience psychosis. When staff see psychotic people behave in this way, they always comment on how unwell they are, however when somebody self-harms in a PICU, nobody thinks they are ill, they just think that they brought it upon themselves and are attention seeking. People admitted for self-harm/suicide are not treated with the same compassion and understanding as how psychotic people are treated. This is a major flaw in the system but it is probably due to the fact that both behaviours are borne from different illnesses and different approaches are needed for both-but still, people should be treated with the same level of kindness. There shouldn't be special empathy for people who are blatantly ill.

Being mentally unwell doesn't have to mean that you strip naked and smear poo everywhere, it could mean that you really struggle with what goes on in your head and you self-destruct.

I'm not just saying this because I'm one of those people who would suffer quietly.

Chapter 28:

Staff Hierarchy

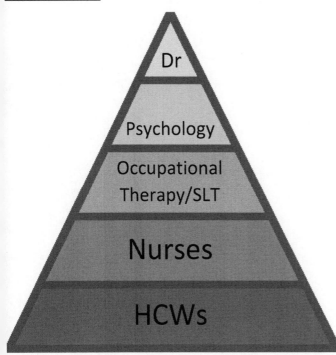

This is the hierarchy of healthcare professionals who are usually are involved with psychiatric inpatient units.

Let's start with the HCWs (Healthcare Worker). Sometimes called CSW (Clinical Support Worker) or HCA (Healthcare Assistant). These are arguably the most important people. HCWs have the most patient contact out of all the hierarchy. Although they do the most work, they rarely get recognition. Many people think they are insignificant and don't matter which is contradictory. It is easy for someone to become an HCW and little qualifications are needed but it is an incredibly difficult job! They go in the "over-worked and underpaid" category. It is their job to serve food, speak to patients, go on observations, ensure sure each need is met. It is actually quite a lot to do. People don't become an HCW for money, it doesn't pay very well and is usually extremely long hours, shifts which can be up to 13 hours. People become HCWs because they like to care for people. These workers get minimal input into decisions around care e.g. discharge or admission. I think of this as manual labour; these workers do the grittiest of jobs for the least amount of money. There are now Nursing Associate roles where HCWs can bridge the gap between HCWs and Nurses. They can dispense meds and do everything an HCW does.

Next up, Nurses. They also fall into the "overworked and underpaid" category. Nurses dispense the medication to patients and it is their job to have 1:1s and write care plans. If something terrible happened to a patient, it would be a nurse who would get the brunt of the consequences, rather than a CSW. Most nurses become nurses because they care. There are very few nurses who come into the profession without compassion. Nurses are in charge of the shift usually. Nurses usually do everything that CSWs do plus more. It is up to these people to share their observations with the clinician on the ward (consultant psychiatrist).

Occupational therapists. I like to think of them as the people who teach you how to live. Most OTs in a psychiatric setting would do cooking or baking with patients. They take you to the bank and on trips out. One of my OTs power walked with me to the bank and took me horse riding, rock climbing and trampolining every week. They help to co-ordinate activities for patients and promote daily living skills or do sensory assessments. They can be really fun.

Speech and Language Therapists usually work with people who have communication difficulties. In mental health settings, it is usually the case where they work with people who have learning difficulties, acquired brain injuries or autism.

Doctors, or Consultant Psychiatrists have the most power when it comes to influencing decisions involving care. They have least patient contact but are expected to know everything about a patient. Not all doctors know what is best. You get good ones and bad ones, much like how you get good and bad people in the world. It is up to luck what pick of the mix you get.

Chapter 29:

Effective practice in Mental Health Care

- Call them service-users not patients. Patients connote that they are controlled by the system. Language is important.
- Person-centred care. Tailor their treatment. Each individual is different and deserves treatment that suits them. It is not a "one-size fits all". This includes adapting your approach to the individual's presentation or communication styles. For example, not all service users will deal well with really boisterous, loud and outgoing people, they may have a more mellow temperament, bear this in mind as this is a prime example of person centred approach with communication styles. Use a personalised treatment package, tailored to the patients' needs. Remember that 2 people with the same diagnosis can act quite differently. For example, any 2 people with autism can be affected very differently.
- Use compassion-focussed and holistic approach. Don't think of service user as a walking mental health illness, we are individuals with a variety of different layers to us. Consider social and environmental factors and not just symptoms. There is more to us than that.
- Decisions around care and treatment should be done *with* us not *to* us! Don't make decisions based purely on your professional opinion. Consult with us first- it is our lives which are going to be affected anyway! Involve service users in each aspect of their care
- My best friend who was diagnosed with psychosis was taken off her anti-psychotics... no, I don't understand their logic either! They didn't consult with her to explain the reason for their decision. Psychiatrists don't need an extensive knowledge, just common sense. They also need an awareness that people's lives are on the line and need to take responsibility that they have a duty to keep people safe first and foremost. If my friend was spoken to about this first, perhaps she might be on the path to recovery sooner.
- Encourage your service user to feel empowered in their care. Encourage them to be a voice of their struggles not a victim of their mental illness. Whilst a nurturing approach in validating their pain is necessary, offering them the victim mentality is not. It will lead to them justifying their risk behaviour and indulging in it more which is ostensibly maladaptive.

- Recovery outcomes need to be looked at and recorded by professionals in order for other practitioners to know what works in the general population in terms of treatment options.
- Evidence-based practice: Look at research on mental health problems and relate to how you can implement this in your practice. There are loads of alternative treatments to different mental illnesses being developed, make the most of them!
- Don't go straight to prescribing meds, this should be a last resort. It should still be used, just sparingly. Putting somebody on meds for the rest of their life will always have some sort of effect. The way I think of it is that meds are like magic and all magic comes with a price. For my friend, she was on anti-psychotics for years and started to have adverse side-effects and started getting severe muscle spasms from it, to the point of needing hospitalisation and experiencing debilitating pain. This is a danger of overmedicating. Putting someone on a cocktail of meds for a sustained period of time will have effects on their physical health and may make them prone to dependency. I know some people really need medication, I know I do. Some doctors tried to tell me that I had an organic psychosis and so I needed m antipsychotics for at least 2-5 years. Some people need medication but there should always be a plan to find alternative ways to helping people, for example, a holistic and therapeutic approach can help like DBT or EMDR. Use psychology, not solely pharmacology. If I was offered intense therapy in my first couple of admissions into hospital, it might have prevented my future problems and risk behaviours because I would have had the skills to deal with it.
- Least restrictive practice. This means that ensuring that the restrictions placed on a service user are as minimal as possible. When I used to self-harm, staff would take away my clothes and strip my room to make it completely sterile. This measure was done to keep me safe from hurting myself. This needed to happen. However, it is good practice to ensure that you are not only helping to maintain a service-user's recovery but also considering their dignity. For example, when I would have self-harm incidents, staff would put me on 1:1 observations (with a staff member being with me at all times) and take everything out of my room. It would have been good practice to put me on 1:1 but only in secluded areas, because that was the only place I would self-harm. This is an example of

- preserving my sense of freedom as much as possible as can be done when sectioned under the Mental Health Act.
- Consider paraphrasing your questions. Ask less questions such as "What's wrong with you?" and more "What has happened to you?" This is not the world of physical health, this is treatment of psychological duress and so should be treated accordingly.
- When it comes to service users who have associated physical health problems, in addition to their mental health condition, consider if their physical health is due to the detriment of their mental wellbeing. In other words, if there is a service user with severe anxiety but also has unexplained physical health systems such as the usual severe stomach pains, think about if the 2 conditions are related. I know for me personally, my eczema and psoriasis got worse when I was having a bad suicidal episode and I had to go on antibiotics. Sometimes the body is telling you what the mind can't.
- Tailor your communication style, especially when working with children and young people. Think: With communication with adolescents; it isn't what you say, it is what they hear. Young people know the social cues and reading between the lines so will know if you are ineffectively communicating.
- Professionals make a lot of mistakes when it comes to treating people. When I was in hospital, my psychiatrist said she wanted to experiment on how I function with being off meds. I became psychotic and would have episodes where I felt like I couldn't control my actions. I was running into walls thinking they were portals, putting my fingers in plugs, thinking they were a portal to another dimension. There was another psychiatrist who gave somebody with bipolar such strong medication, that it was over the legally safe limit of antipsychotics and lithium, this girl ended up being manic for weeks, if not months. Other health professionals lied to me about my diagnosis, saying I was bipolar but never thought of telling me until I discovered this in my notes, years later. I was told by professionals that I was unwell and needed psychotics to which another health person would then tell me that I was faking psychosis.

Point is, nobody is perfect-doctors, nurses, and therapists...don't always know what is wrong. Don't be afraid to question their judgment, if that is what your treatment requires, then do so. Every professional will have a different opinion based upon their experiences and interpretation. Mental health is never black and white- I learned that the hard way. Factor this in when thinking about your recovery.

<u>Safeguarding</u>

In regards to safeguarding, professionals need to be more vigilant and mindful of the lengths people will go in order to kill themselves. For example, when I was in the community and ingested items, the crisis team were called once I was deemed physically medically fit and they spoke to me. I told them I was fine and was not going to kill myself so they discharged me however this led to me running into moving traffic so I was sectioned again. Safety is key when dealing with mental health problems. It should always come first, even if it is against the person's wishes. For example, when I was suicidal, it was always something professionals had to hand over in order to keep me safe, even if I didn't want other knowing. This was because if I managed to follow through with my intentions, then the person I confided in would be responsible for not effectively safeguarding me.

Chapter 30:

Co-Production with Youth participation:

In the world of mental health, co-production or service user involvement is the new big thing. Youth participation in mental health is the new black, it is what all good services are using these days! What co-production means is including service users in the development of future mental health services.

Why co-production is a good thing:

Who else knows best how to run or change a service than the people who have been through it themselves? We are called Experts by Experience and the name couldn't be more fitting! We are specialists in mental health affairs. Not only does it benefit the EbE's but it also gives the health professionals an insight which one wouldn't be aware of, without experiencing.

Characteristics of Genuine Co-production:

- Not tokenistic but an authentic engagement with mutual respect of both the young person and the professional.
- Avoid medical technical jargon as it can undermine the power and equity imbalance of the young person and professional. It is already anxiety-provoking being in the same room as people who have masters and doctorates, let alone when they start using words you don't understand.
- Ground rules should always be set in advance and in collaboration with the group, outlining confidentiality, respecting people, giving everyone a chance to speak and maintain candour in a polite way.
- Giving as much information before hand as possible.
- Offering debriefs to the service user if the activity that is being co-produced is distressing.

Chapter 31:

Pursuit of Superficial Nature:

Happiness is not an enduring feeling. It is a fleeting moment of overwhelming elation or subtle contentment. It is an emotion that, like sadness, is not lasting. Pursuing happiness should not be your aim in life because it isn't a long term goal. Eventually happiness will be replaced with another emotion. It is good to do things that make you happy but I wouldn't recommend that you actively seek just that. The aim in life should be about pursuing purpose. This will naturally breed happiness and contentment. My purpose is to help others. I do this by my mental health advocacy work and helping people to access services so that they don't have to get to the point I got to. I fulfil my purpose by working hard towards being a neuroscientist in order to find cures and do research on disorders that people don't usually think of.

Purpose helps with acceptance of the state of being and that things will be difficult at times and things will be great at other times. It is being grateful for what you already have.

Years of being unhappy and unwell has made me realise this. It has meant I have been able to build a life worth living.

Chapter 32:

Battle Scars

I have self-harm scars. I don't want to get rid of them. Why? Why would I willingly want to keep a remainder of the pain I have been through?

Yes, I have self-harm scars, some permanent and deep. I choose not to have laser treatment or cover them up with make up because I am not ashamed of them. They show how strong I am now. They represent empowerment of me being a warrior of the battle with my own mind.

My scars show the struggle I went through in order to fight for a life worth living. Showing my scars doesn't symbolise being proud of self-harm or promoting it, but the opposite, accepting struggle for what it is and striving for wellness.

Life isn't about the struggle, but about how you get back up from the struggle.

Chapter 33:

Belonging

The place I felt like I most belonged was in hospital. Everybody in hospital usually matures quickly due to the nature of their struggles. The suffering people go through with mental illness is pure hardship. Most young people don't understand the extent of the kinds of suffering that happens in life. The most affliction they would have felt is people ignoring them on snapchat. I have had people talking to me about how bad they thought their life was because their schoolbag broke. No, that isn't a bad life. There are worse things that happen in the world. For example, young people suffering with their traumatic past and who are held down on the floor by 5 people in order to give them an injection of anti-psychotic medication to stop their voices in their head. Suffering is being tube fed because you won't eat because you think people are going to poison your food. Suffering is being transferred to a psychiatric unit 150 miles away from your home in order to receive treatment for your chronic suicidality. Worse things happen in life, but most people live a sheltered life and don't realise this.

Despite all the bad things that happened in hospital, it was one of the few places that gave me validation and unconditional care. This was why I felt like I belonged.

Chapter 34:

People I am proud of:

Too often, people forget to think of the ones other than themselves. I am guilty of this. I am proud of the following people:

A middle aged man with learning disabilities is the longest living survivor of his rare illness. He cracks me up big time. He has learning disabilities and he is soooooo cute. He always shakes your hand when you meet him and then holds onto your hand.

He thinks he is a business man and goes around everywhere with a briefcase in his hand. In the briefcase, is a wad of paper that he stole from the staff office with random pamphlets and leaflets! He gives these to other people to read and sign (I'm telling you, one day, you will sign your life away to him and you will regret it!).

Sometimes he grabs his phone (which has no battery in it) and he pretends he is speaking to his mum. He does this when he is upset, pretends to speak to his mum, who actually died years ago but after he finishes talking, he feels better. If that works for him, that's great, but it is still sad to know.

He loves chocolate and had 3 chocolate bars at a time but his support worker said, "You're diabetic, you can't eat all that chocolate! What else would you like?" He replied, "Ok, then. Can I have a diabetic burger?" He is too much!

One time, he went to general hospital and the doctors were telling him that he was fine to go home and he needed to go, they were discharging him. He subsequently rang up the manager of the home and said to bring up 2 pairs of trousers because he was "staying the night"...! What?! Funny man. Eventually, the hospital staff told him he had to go or they would call security to which he replied, "Don't worry, I will be back!" He is an absolute joker but doesn't realise it!

Chapter 35:

During my time in hospital, I have made numerous nominations for the staff who worked with me, here are some of them.

Psychologist Nomination:

Linda is a psychologist, works in a Low Secure CAMHS unit for mentally ill adolescents who require a long term inpatient provision. Linda works with these vulnerable young people and has an imperative role in helping with psychological treatment. She is a counselling psychologist, recently qualified for her Master's degree. On a day to day basis, she works with individuals to aid them in their journey to recovery. I was a patient here and she changed my life.

I never would have thought she would have such an impact on me and that I would come to love them. It took months for me to trust her and get to know them, but she was patient, more patient that they had ever been in any other unit and I have been in 7 other units, all over the UK. My psychologist never gave up on me, even when my psychiatrist just wanted to send me to an all-autistic residential in a few months.

Linda is worthy of an award because of her sheer determination and passion for young people's mental wellbeing. When I was at Hillview Hospital, I was in a dark place, engaging in suicidal behaviour and, in hindsight, meeting Linda was the best thing that could have happened to me. She nurtured me and worked with me, meeting me every week without fail for nearly a year. Unlike most psychologists she never gave up on me, despite my hostile attitude towards her. Linda took the time to understand me, looking past my walls that I had built so high, after years of being in and out of psychiatric institutions. She was one of the few people who never gave up on me. Her relentless persistence is admirable, her unwavering vigour to help people is refreshing to see. After 4 years of being in the mental health system, I have come to observe how professionals around me work and how to tell if someone genuinely wants to help and I can honestly say; Linda has the purest of intentions. After 4 months of her making a tremendous effort to encourage me to engage, I began psychological work with her every week twice a week for 7 months. Together, we went through my past, opening my allegorical "can of worms" and Linda would skilfully help me close it again. We went through schema therapy and helped to identify my maladaptive schemas, core beliefs based off past experiences, as well as coping skills for the future. Finally here I am, the most well I have been since I was 11. I am now going to college, doing my GCSEs, looking at supported community accommodation and engaging in projects to improve future mental health services. This is all thanks to Linda. It was Linda who constantly reminded me to utilise my skills. Nursing staff would support me, but it was in Psychology where the real grit was. My gratitude towards her is boundless. She has saved my life. If I had not met her, I probably would have entered adult services and been in hospital for a lot longer than I have been. She has worked with me to prevent my revolving-door-patient cycle and has transformed how I view myself, others and life I general, completely altering my once-negative attitude to the world. Without her, I wouldn't be alive today.

I remember when I first started engaging properly with her, she said that no matter how hard it would be, I could tell her anything and she would be able to be strong enough for the both of us. Linda was the only psychologist who didn't yield in the face of hardship. I cry tears on sadness and joy when I think of this-sadness because I know that I may never see her again after working with her so closely, but also joy, because of how much she has changed my life. When I first met her, I said that I had a predisposition to disliking people called Linda because an old psychologist called Linda had a calamity occur to her. In the face of hostility, borne from the nature of my mental illness, she continued to work with me and wasn't in the least bit fazed.

But why Linda, you ask? What is so special about her? Linda worked overtime, she would come into work at 7:30 am and leave at around 7:30 pm when her job was simply 9-5. She consistently over exerted her efforts, going above and beyond to secure a future for the people she worked with. Yes, it may have been her job, but she is a pioneer, an Einstein in wealth of scientific and psychology-based knowledge, a Mahatma Ghandi in the care of her patients and a Martin Luther King in her resolve to fight for what is right.

Very few mental health professionals receive recognition for their efforts and are told thank you, despite how rewarding their work is. She is overworked and under-recognised. In consideration of the difficult aspects there are of being a mental health practitioner, she has managed to remain unfalteringly professional whilst still showing her compassion. I am indebted to her and I am sure many others feel the same way. She deserves to be paid in glory.

(Got the OT to join because why not?)

Occupational Therapist, Helen's supporting statement: I have worked alongside Linda, within an MDT capacity and could not think of a better suited candidate for this award. As detailed in the nomination, Linda often goes over and beyond for the young people within our care and will always ensure their opinions, wants and needs are considered within meetings. Linda always takes a "can do" approach and nothing is too much effort for her within her job role. All Young People within our care have a positive relationship with Linda, and as detailed she will always ensure that time is taken to encourage the Young People to fully engage with any psychological work required. Within Hillview Hospital, we as a team can be presented with challenging situations which require additional support, time and effort to be spent with the Young People and staffing team. Linda will always volunteer to assist with these matters when she is available and has been noted to work outside of her working hours to ensure a high level of quality care is provided to all Young People. Linda has been noted to include a multitude of different therapies within her practice and will willingly adapt sessions to suit the individual. Linda has been noted to always take a person centred holistic approach to all care provided.

Linda not only supports the Young People in their care, but also promotes and empowers the whole team, both MDT and Support Workers to fulfil their job roles to the best of their ability. She has been noted to give the staff time to debrief and attend reflective practice sessions in order to discuss any concerns they have and to improve this within their own future practice. Linda has introduced a wide range of psychometric assessments to inform the patient care. Linda has also implemented new group therapy sessions such as Carousel and the Smile project within Hillview Hospital, which have been a success with our Young People.

(And the nurse who is ma bish:)

I have known and worked alongside Linda Grey-Thomas as a work colleague within the Multi-disciplinary team since assuming my Nursing post here at Hillview in March, 2018. This period so mentioned has been the busiest the service has been through since inception due to several factors amongst which are acuity, service restructure, regulators scrutiny and Management reform. This level of pressure meant that the MDT were required to pull resources together and go well and above their job role & scope of practice in order to maintain the level of care standard required, as well as meet regulatory requirements. "Above scope of practice" is used within this context to denote when additional sets of skills outside one's discipline were called to use.

The above brief introduction is necessary for the following reasons: (a) it offers some sort of insight on the level of commitment and flexibility that Linda must have exhibited within these period and (b) an explanation on why I consider myself in a position to nominate Linda for this award.

Although my background is Nursing, Linda has been a great source of knowledge and I have come to learn a lot of transferable skills from her. I'm therefore delighted to support this application made by Ms Sohawon and nominate Linda for the following reasons:

Linda's ability to easily establish trust and build therapeutic relationship with young people who are in crisis are exceptional. Her calm demeanour creates a positive presence and promotes therapeutic approach within the Nursing team.

Within the MDT, Linda has been inspirational in promoting healthy debate that instigate challenge to clinical practices. Similarly, Linda is a strong advocate to evidence-based interventions and least restrictive practice.

Her knowledge on each young person's clinical background, social circumstances as well as their prognosis has personally inspired and helped me during professional meetings and Tribunals.

Her flexible approach to the demands of the service is constantly being talked about with the Nursing team. From organising the young people's forum to running staff reflective practice, Linda would put in additional unpaid hours to ensure people's views are heard, needs are met, staff morals are lifted, people feel supported and appreciated. Of all these, my biggest learning point which currently influence my approach is her ability to remain calm in a difficult and stressful situation.

With her broad knowledge and skills that cuts across all areas of clinical practice to day to day operational running of the service, Linda has been actively involved in helping the service pull through a difficult time last year. She is also actively involved in various committees tasked to improve service whilst still carrying her Psychology caseloads and delivering these to an exceptionally high standard. Needless to mention the major impact her Psychology sessions have had on the young people. Evidence of these lies on the frequent discharges and referrals to stepdown facility as well as nominations especially to this merit award from a young person and colleagues. As a registered Nurse, I strongly subscribe to a recovery/psychology model as opposed to pharmacology. I have and continue to consult with Linda on 'cases that challenge my knowledge and perception'. And without doubt both my Nursing colleagues and I have always benefitted from Linda's support and knowledge.

I strongly recommend Linda for this award of merit, for all her efforts to young people's recovery as well as commitments to the service

Emmanuel Nomination:

When I was in my Low Secure Unit, I met an excellent, devoted and hard-working nurse whom I grew to become fond of and seek support from. Once I was discharged, I nominated for a nursing award from the Royal College of Nursing. This is what I wrote:

Emmanuel has contributed greatly to the delivery of care given in the Mental Health nursing sector. His skillset exceeds that of being "just a good nurse". His innovative ideas has had a dramatically positive impact on my life, as his patient.

I was admitted to a Low Secure Unit for a year, beginning January 2018. From March onwards, my Named Nurse was allocated as Emmanuel. Little did I know that this was going to be the best thing to have happened to me...

I was shown empathy, patience and never ending diligence. His manner of mansuetude, consistent integrity and high standard of professionalism eased me into my journey to recovery. From May, I began therapeutically engaging and Emmanuel did not once feign in his perseverance to help me strive towards mental stability, even in the face of relapse. He had an outstanding understanding of my diagnosis and was mindful of it during the time we worked together.

However, it wasn't just the fact of being an excellent nurse, it was his original and slightly unconventional ideology of introducing coping strategies into my life through encouraging me to utilise fitness and I began to attend the hospital's gym facilities with Emmanuel's recommendation. Within a matter of months, I used exercise as an antidepressant and have continued to use it since. This heavily influenced my improved mental state.

Now I have stepped down from Low Secure and am moving on in my life. I went from being psychotic and tying a suspended ligature to having unescorted leave with my family for the first time in 2 years, having firmly established coping strategies and being on the verge of discharge.

Emmanuel once told me it isn't about *reacting* to suicide attempts, it's about being *proactive* in stopping someone from feeling suicidal in the first place. It was his contributions that brought my out of the darkness and crafted me into the resilient and empowered individual I am today. I am walking and breathing evidence of his extensive efforts and dedication to the Royal College of Nurses and the mental health sector.

(This is what my Daddy-O had written:)

This nurse has saved my daughter's life. He encouraged her to achieve recovery in a way that I, as a parent, never could. He kept me informed of changes in her care, unlike many nurses have done so in the past. His innovative and forward-thinking nature has significantly impacted on the quality of my daughter's life. My gratitude is boundless.

Emmanuel always encouraged Zaynab (my daughter) to use fitness to improve her mental health. Without this, my daughter wouldn't be where she is now; engaging with therapeutic interventions, working towards recovery and on the verge of being discharged from inpatient CAMHS.

He always took the time to explain exactly what difficulties were perpetuating my daughter's mental illness and how best to approach her. In all $3_{1/2}$ years of having my daughter in hospital, no nurse has been so dedicated. For 30 minutes at a time, we would have detailed conversations regarding my daughter's treatment plan. In my experience, very few nurses have done this. He would always have time for me, despite his busy schedule.

As a parent, it is nerve-racking to have a child placed under a section under professional care with little information and understanding. Emmanuel educated me as to how best to help my daughter as well as offering me moral support. It is difficult for both the family and the person undergoing mental illness and Emmanuel seemed to understand this really well. Many past professionals overlooked this.

Emmanuel is a pioneer of his field, introducing ground-breaking research of how exercise benefits mental health. He presents with incredible interpersonal skills, consideration and humility.

I hold him in high esteem for kick-starting my daughter's road to recovery.

(I roped in my fave OT and Boss of a psychologist to write some stuff for ma homie, Emmanuel☺

I support this application from witnessing and working alongside Emmanuel as an RMN. Emmanuel takes pride and time in ensuring that he provides high quality care for all the Young People detained under the Mental Health Act within our service. Emmanuel is able to advocate the young person's request as well as support the clinical team in ensuring the best decision is made for the young people within our care. Emmanuel demonstrates excellent skills within his nursing practice and effectively communicates with all the young people and his staffing team.

Emmanuel effectively supports the young people within his care when they express their difficulties. He is innovative and able to express various coping strategies which can be implemented immediately to support the young people. As previously detailed, where appropriate Emmanuel encourages the use of physical activity within a young person's care and treatment which has demonstrated evident benefits.

Emmanuel continues to excel within his field of practice and continually puts the young person at the forefront of their care. He has an excellent manner with the young people and maintains positive therapeutic relationships.

I am delighted to support this application made by Miss Sohawon. I have had the pleasure of working with Emmanuel since he joined No View in 2018 and witness his professionalism, dedication, hard-working and motivational manner in which he carries out all of his work. Emmanuel has a gift of being able to reach patients who have built their defences so high, that they will not allow others in, but with his patience and gentle nature he is able to build a trusting and therapeutic relationship with them.

Emmanuel always ensures that he makes time to spend with the patients and it is clear that he is very passionate about his work. Nothing ever seems too much trouble for him, and he is happy to think of new ways to engage a young person and draw on his own experiences to support them to achieve their goals. During Review meetings, Manager Hearings and Tribunals, Emmanuel ensures that he advocates for the young person and makes strenuous efforts to ensure that a fair presentation of each young person is delivered with their needs at the core of all his reports and work.

As part of the wider MDT, Emmanuel is a very valued member of the team. He supports all disciplines and encourages the young people to attend all sessions and views a holistic treatment plan as vital to achieve the best outcomes for the each young person. Emmanuel is very conscientious and a team player, always willing to offer advice and support to colleagues when needed.

Personally, I hold Emmanuel in high regard and believe that he is a credit to the nursing profession and is very worthy of this nomination.

Dr P Nomination:

Dr P has gone above and beyond the normal. I have been in mental health services for 4 years and she is one of the few consultants who listens to what I say and validates my feelings. She has come to understand me very much. She is humble and has time for me unlike most consultant psychiatrists I have met. When I was struggling, I asked for her to speak to me and apologised for seeing her multiple times in the same week, to which she replied, "Even if you have to see me 500 times a day, I don't mind, as long as you're OK." No doctor has said this to me before and I have been to 5 different hospitals all over the UK.

She understands the complex nature of my mental health so well and has taken the time to get to know me, not just my illness. I have seen her go home at 7:30 at times which shows how hard working she is. I produced a show called the Craziest Showman based off of the Greatest Showman with staff to play the characters and she attended rehearsals with genuine eagerness and enthusiasm.

She deserves this award because not many mental health professionals are recognised for their efforts and she is an outstanding doctor as well as an altruistic person. Her compassion is boundless and this is blatantly evident through her actions and efforts. She needs to know that her hard work has not gone unnoticed. Her integrity and perseverance are much appreciated.

She is a merit to the NHS system and I am blessed to have her as my doctor.

Phase 3: Miscellaneous Awakenings

Chapter 36:

How Do I Learn How To Live: From the Story of an Ex-Suicidal?

I have been suicidal since I was 14-for 4 years, so most of my adolescent-hood. I always made plans and attempts to end my life on every birthday. I had no idea I would make it this far in life. It makes me think that I put so much time, so much efforts in ending my life that I feel I don't know what to do now that I want to live it. My purpose for most of my teenage years was to die. Now I am out of the darkness, I don't know what to do, there's a whole world out there waiting for me- there's just so much to do and it's overwhelming. I can go travelling, get a doctorate, and protest for women's rights...the list is endless.

When one is stuck in psychiatric institutions, one forgets how great real life is. People who get admitted always say about how they want to be out but when asked "What would you do?" they are often speechless.

In preparation for each birthday, I would write letters addressed to people I knew, invitations to my funeral. I would put "Ding Dong! The bitch is dead. Marvel at the Borderlines. Bye, Felicia!" (At which point, everybody would instinctively ask "Who is Felicia?" to which I would face-palm and reply, "Urban dictionary it!")

That was my template for my suicide notes, which I would call "deposits of my packages of pain"...but then there was the funeral planning.

I would plan that I would have my funeral at school because that was the only place where I felt a sense of belonging. My favourite teachers would be there, all my favourite staff members from all the different hospitals I had been to, my best friends and a few family members. I used to write out invitations to my funeral to all those people, not to mention writing my own will which would say that half of all my money would go to charity (I could never decide between WaterAid or a mental health charity like Mind) and that my organs could be donated to research. My will would be pages long. I considered giving it to my solicitor (who represented me at my mental health tribunals, but obviously this might raise alarm bells...)

My plans for actually killing myself would be scarily detailed and quite morbid. I wouldn't just make the one plan, no, I would make contingency plans. I would have plans from Plan A to Plan F.

When I was ill, I used to think of life in a very pessimistic way. I had no will to live. Here is a snippet of my personal diary:

"In the cold clockworks of the stars and the nations, the warping of the space continuum, and the depths of natural galaxies (as humans), we are, in all candour, significantly insignificant, burdened with idle purpose. We are ailed with internal suffering. I am not fooled by the façade of hope, nor the mirage of a future. "

I also made analogies of Narnia which in my mind, meant Heaven. I thought that "I was meant to go to Narnia. It is natural. If it wasn't natural, I wouldn't be thinking it. So wanting to go somewhere like Narnia isn't an anomalous desire.

With every fibre of my being, I so desperately wanted to die. I think the only thing that stopped me was being in hospital because I knew that it is less likely that a suicide in a psychiatric unit would be possible. It isn't unheard of but a lot less likely.

After a year of therapy (schema, CBT and DBT), I am out of the suicidality cycle. I have things I look forward to and am blessed to have some really good people in my life.

Ya gal, ya boi ZeZe is discharged!!! ZeZe is out, released!

Bye Felicia, Bye Sheniqua, Bye Moniqua! A bish is done with psych wards.

Chapter 37:

The Bird's Nest

The birds nest is my supported living placement, where I live.

The staff there are so funny.

Kaden, the staff member, reminds me constantly of the world's best wonder tonic for any ailment known- humour. Ursila who is obsessed with kebabs. Brianna taught me important lessons about friends: you don't need them, you want them. I enjoy our deep chats about my past. Henrietta talking every time you see her for at least 25 minutes at a time minimum. Sheena always talks about wanting to lose weight but the longest she can go without eating take away is 2 days. Charlotte, another staff member makes me giggle, I think she was born into the wrong culture. She is a white person on the outside but a brown person on the inside. She knows all the Pakistani lingo- "tutti" for "poo" and "behta" for "darling".

There is a service user who catches any spiders she finds and chases staff around with them. She has a specific spider container. She also goes behind staff members' backs and unclips their bra in public. Another service user is an old 65 year old man and all he talks about is taking drugs and having a "spliff". Once the smell of weed spread into my lounge and I (in my naivety) thought it was a drain problem. On the third floor. Yes, well done, me.

The registered manager and deputy are my best friends, they love me and they know me so well. I call my manager my "registered mommy" instead of "registered manager". She is the best manager I could have asked for. The deputy is there for me, always. She said that even after I have left my supported living, she will still want to be in touch with me, I love her unconditionally for being there for me. We have a running joke where the 2 managers are allowed to say anything they want, that they might get in trouble for but they have to say "without prejudice". Without prejudice means you can say something to someone but if the listener later discloses what was said, the person who spoke can legally deny saying that so nobody is held accountable.

I have my own individual apartment with a kitchen, bedroom, bathroom and living room. Staff keep my kitchen knives and medication because that is something I need support with managing. Outside my flat, is a hall which leads to the communal area which is a lounge where the staff are if I ever need them. There is a staff member there 24/7 and there are night shift workers. I have a set of number of hours of support, so I get 6 hours of 1:1 support each which is quite intensive but it is spread out throughout the week.

I am now in College doing a levels, Biology, Chemistry and Psychology. I do public speaking at universities, corporate fundraisers and conferences about experience of mental health. My next steps are to go to University and do a degree in neuroscience, biochemistry or psychotherapy. I want a career in scientific research and hopefully can do research on topics of mental health of which there is little literature about for example, Complex PTSD (Post Traumatic Stress Disorder) and my illness, BPD (Borderline Personality Disorder).

 My journey to independence will be through moving in my second year at university once I am ready.

I want to go travelling around the world, firstly to the Aurora Borealis, Northern lights and to see the Large CERN Hadron Collider.

I have found purpose- I want to devote my life to helping people. When I don't want to help myself, I can still help someone else.

From running into walls, thinking they were portals, here I am today, doing lectures at universities on my experience of CAMHS, talking publicly about my struggles, going to college, having independent access to the community (something I haven't had in 4 years)...I have built a life worth living. I just want to paint the universe with rainbows!

I now do pubic speaking at conferences, corporate fundraisers, universities... all about my past struggles. I am now the most well I have been since the age of 11. If I hadn't gone through all the things that have happened, I wouldn't be where I am today. It is a great day to be alive!

I could flee into the darkness. I could let the shadows welcome me back home, let them hijack the reins to my life. No, I'm tired of running from hospital to hospital.

~~It's time to go back home.~~ I am home.

Acknowledgments:

I would like to thank the following people for pushing me to be the best version of myself.

Thanks to my dad and mum for always trying to be there for me and being pro-active in advising me to build my future.

Thanks to H and B at Presh for loving me unconditionally.

Thanks to everyone in all my hospitals, especially Rochelle, Sick Boi, Jordie, Nate, Preetstick, Benny, Leeam, Alice, Jimbo, Fiddle, Ellabella, Hazelle, Sammy, Kez, Linnie.

Thanks to my educational institutions for believing in me; KEVI Handsworth, Highclare, James Brindley and Cadbury. Staff, you know who you are.

About the Author:

Zaynab Sohawon who goes by the alias of ZeZe Jones is an 18 year old. This book was written by her to encapture the journey she has been on of being sectioned for 4 years in psychiatric inpatient services.

Despite having Emotionally Unstable Personality Disorder, autism and more, ZeZe has channelled her inner resilience to share her experience to prevent other young people from getting to the low point she got to.

Now she works with co-production steering groups as an Expert by Experience to affect change in the mental health system as well as advising on youth mental health research in universities.

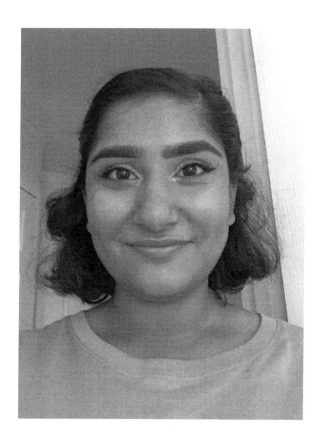

Printed in Poland
by Amazon Fulfillment
Poland Sp. z o.o., Wrocław

54571527R00072